Environmental Health Criteria 132

TRICHLORFON

First draft prepared by Dr J. Sekizawa, Dr M. Takeda and Dr K. Matsumoto (National Institute of Hygienic Sciences, Japan) and Dr M. Eto (Kyushu University, Japan), with the assistance of Dr J. Miyamoto and Dr M. Matsuo (Sumitomo Chemical Company)

World Health Organization
Geneva, 1992

The **International Programme on Chemical Safety (IPCS)** is a joint venture of the United Nations Environment Programme, the International Labour Organisation, and the World Health Organization. The main objective of the IPCS is to carry out and disseminate evaluations of the effects of chemicals on human health and the quality of the environment. Supporting activities include the development of epidemiological, experimental laboratory, and risk-assessment methods that could produce internationally comparable results, and the development of manpower in the field of toxicology. Other activities carried out by the IPCS include the development of know-how for coping with chemical accidents, coordination of laboratory testing and epidemiological studies, and promotion of research on the mechanisms of the biological action of chemicals.

WHO Library Cataloguing in Publication Data

Trichlorfon.

(Environmental health criteria ; 132)

1.Trichlorfon - poisoning 2.Trichlorfon - toxicity 3. Environmental exposure I.Series

ISBN 92 4 157132 2 (NLM Classification: WA 240)
ISSN 0250-863X

Printed in Finland

92/9011 Rev 1 — Vammala — 5500

CONTENTS

ENVIRONMENTAL HEALTH CRITERIA FOR TRICHLORFON

WHO TASK GROUP ON ENVIRONMENTAL HEALTH CRITERIA FOR TRICHLORFON AND FENITROTHION

Members

Dr V. Benes, Department of Toxicology and Reference Laboratory, Institute of Hygiene and Epidemiology, Prague, Czech and Slovak Federal Republic

Dr C. Carrington, Division of Toxicological Review and Evaluation, Food and Drug Administration, Washington DC, USA (*Joint Rapporteur*)

Dr W. Dedek, Department of Chemical Toxicology Academic of Sciences, Leipzig, Germany

Dr S. Dobson, Institute of Terrestrial Ecology, Monks Wood Experimental Station, Huntingdon, United Kingdom

Dr D.J. Ecobichon, Department of Pharmacology and Therapeutics, McGill University, Montreal, Canada

Dr M. Eto, Department of Agricultural Chemistry, Kyushu University, Fukuoka-shi, Japan (*Vice-Chairman)*

Dr Bo Holmstedt, Department of Toxicology, Swedish Medical Research Council, Karolinska Institute, Stockholm, Sweden

Dr S.K. Kashyap, National Institute of Occupational Health, Ahmedabad, India

Dr J. Miyamoto, Takarazuka Research Centre, Hyogo, Japan

Dr H. Spencer, United States Environmental Protection Agency, Washington DC, USA (*Chairman)*

Dr M. Takeda, National Institute of Hygienic Sciences, Tokyo, Japan

Observers

Dr M. Matsuo, Biochemistry and Toxicology Laboratory, Sumitomo Chemical Co. Ltd, Osaka-shi, Japan (representing GIFAP)

Secretariat

Dr J. Sekizawa, National Institute of Hygienic Sciences, Tokyo, Japan (*Joint Rapporteur)*

Dr K.W. Jager, IPCS, World Health Organization, Geneva, Switzerland (*Secretary)*

NOTE TO READERS OF THE CRITERIA DOCUMENTS

Every effort has been made to present information in the criteria documents as accurately as possible without unduly delaying their publication. In the interest of all users of the Environmental Health Criteria documents, readers are kindly requested to communicate any errors that may have occurred to the Director of the International Programme on Chemical Safety, World Health Organization, Geneva, Switzerland, in order that they may be included in corrigenda, which will appear in subsequent volumes.

* * *

A detailed data profile and a legal file can be obtained from the International Register of Potentially Toxic Chemicals, Palais des Nations, 1211 Geneva 10, Switzerland (Telephone no. 7988400 - 7985850).

ENVIRONMENTAL HEALTH CRITERIA FOR TRICHLORFON AND FENITROTHION

A WHO Task Group on Environmental Health Criteria for Trichlorfon and Fenitrothion met at the World Health Organization, Geneva, from 10 to 14 December 1990. Dr K.W. Jager, IPCS, welcomed the participants on behalf of Dr M. Mercier, Director of the IPCS, and the three IPCS cooperating organizations (UNEP/ILO/WHO). The Group reviewed and revised the drafts and made evaluations of the risks for human health and the environment from exposure to trichlorfon and fenitrothion.

The first draft of the EHC on trichlorfon was prepared collaboratively by Dr M. Eto of the Kyushu University, Dr J. Miyamoto and Dr M. Matsuo of the Sumitomo Chemical Company, and Dr M. Takeda and Dr K. Matsumoto of the National Institute of Hygienic Sciences of Japan. The scientific editing was performed by Dr J. Sekizawa of the National Institute of Hygienic Sciences of Japan. Dr K.W. Jager of the International Programme on Chemical Safety, assisted in the preparation of the second draft, incorporating comments received following the circulation of the first drafts to the IPCS contact points for Environmental Health Criteria documents.

Dr K.W. Jager of the IPCS Central Unit was responsible for the scientific content of the documents, and Mrs M.O. Head of Oxford for the editing.

The fact that Sumitomo Chemical Company Limited, Japan (trichlorfon and fenitrothion) and Bayer AG, Germany (trichlorfon) made available to the IPCS and the Task Group their proprietary toxicological information on the products under discussion is gratefully acknowledged. This allowed the Task Group to make its evaluation on the basis of more complete data.

The efforts of all who helped in the preparation and finalization of the documents are gratefully acknowledged.

INTRODUCTION

The major transformation product of trichlorfon in mammals, including human beings, is dichlorvos, the cholinesterase inhibiting activity of which is at least 100 times that of trichlorfon (Hofer, 1981). Trichlorfon can be said to act in the mammalian body as a "slow release source" for dichlorvos, which may be of essential importance for, among others, its schistosomicidal effect (Nordgren, 1981; Nordgren et al., 1978).

Only information directly related to trichlorfon will be discussed and evaluated in this publication.

For an evaluation of the health and environmental hazards of dichlorvos, the reader should refer to EHC No. 79: Dichlorvos (WHO, 1989). A more complete treatise on the effects of organophosphorus insecticides in general, especially their short- and long-term effects on the nervous system, and their treatment, can be found in EHC No. 63: *Organophosphorus insecticides - A general introduction* (WHO, 1986).

A comprehensive review of Russian literature up to 1983, on the toxicity and hazards of trichlorfon, has been published by the International Register of Potentially Toxic Chemicals (IRPTC/GKNT, 1983).

1. SUMMARY AND EVALUATION, CONCLUSIONS, AND RECOMMENDATIONS

1.1 Summary and evaluation

1.1.1 Exposure

Trichlorfon is an organophosphorus insecticide that has been in use since the early 1950s. In agriculture, it is mainly used against insect pests in field and fruit crops. Trichlorfon is also used to control forest insects and for the control of parasites in domestic animals. Under the name of metrifonate, trichlorfon is used for the treatment of human infestation by *Schistosoma haematobium*. It is considered to be a slow release reservoir of dichlorvos. Trichlorfon is available in the form of an emulsifiable concentrate, powder, dust, granules, a solution, and ultra-low volume concentrates.

The air concentration of trichlorfon insecticide may be as high as 0.1 mg/m^3, soon after spraying, but levels decrease within days to below 0.01 mg/m^3. Levels of trichlorfon in run-off water from sprayed areas may be as high as 50 μg/litre, though levels in surface waters are usually much lower and decrease rapidly.

Trichlorfon degrades rapidly in soil, and levels generally decrease to negligible amounts within one month of application. It is relatively stable in water below pH 5.5. At higher pH, trichlorfon is transformed to dichlorvos. While microorganisms and plants may metabolize trichlorfon, the most important route of removal is abiotic hydrolysis.

With a few exceptions, levels of trichlorfon on crops are below 10 mg/kg the day after application, and fall to below 0.1 mg/kg during the two weeks following.

Milk from cows treated with trichlorfon for pest control may contain residues as high as 1.2 mg/litre 2 h after application, but the levels decline to below 0.1 mg/litre 24 h after treatment. Significant levels of trichlorfon have not been found in meat from treated animals. Eggs from treated hens have been found to contain 0.05 mg trichlorfon/kg.

1.1.2 *Uptake, metabolism, and excretion*

Trichlorfon is readily absorbed via all routes of exposure (oral, dermal, inhalation) and is rapidly distributed to the tissues of the body. Peak blood concentrations were detected within 1-2 h, almost total disappearance from the blood stream occurring in a matter of 1.5-4 h. The biological half-life of trichlorfon in the mammalian blood was estimated to be in the range of 30 min.

Trichlorfon undergoes transformation to dichlorvos (2,2-dichlorovinyl dimethyl phosphate), via dehydrochlorination, in water, biological fluids, and tissues, at pH values higher than 5.5. Dichlorvos is the physiologically active anticholinesterase. The main routes of degradation are demethylation, P-C bond cleavage, and ester hydrolysis via dichlorvos. The major metabolites of trichlorfon found *in vivo* are demethyl trichlorfon, demethyl dichlorvos, dimethyl hydrogen phosphate, methyl hydrogen phosphate, phosphoric acid, and trichloroethanol. The last metabolite is found in the urine as a glucuronide conjugate.

Trichlorfon and metabolic products are primarily eliminated via the urine. Studies conducted with radiolabelled (^{14}C-methyl and ^{32}P-) trichlorfon revealed that the bulk of the chemical was eliminated in the form of water-soluble material, little being chloroform-soluble. Some 66-70% of the water-soluble products appeared in the urine within 12 h while 24% of the ^{14}C-methyl material was eliminated in the expired air as carbon dioxide (CO_2). Low levels of trichlorfon and metabolites have been detected in bovine milk following oral and dermal treatment of the animals.

1.1.3 *Effects on organisms in the environment*

Trichlorfon is moderately toxic for fish (96-h LC_{50} values range between 0.45 mg/litre and 51 mg/litre) and moderately to highly toxic for aquatic arthropods (48-h/96-h LC_{50} values range between 0.75 μg/litre and 7800 μg/litre). However, reported concentrations of trichlorfon in surface waters, after application in forests at 6 kg/ha, fall short of these ranges. Thus, in normal usage, trichlorfon will have little or no effect on populations of aquatic organisms, since other groups, such as molluscs and microorganisms are less sensitive than arthropods. LD_{50} values from laboratory studies ranging from 40 mg/kg to 180 mg/kg indicate that trichlorfon is moderately toxic for birds. However, in field studies, no effects on numbers, breeding pairs, nesting success, or mortality of forest songbirds were seen following aerial application of trichlorfon. An observed reduction in singing and increased feeding activity may have been the result of a reduction in food organisms. There is no indication that trichlorfon will adversely affect organisms in the terrestrial environment, other than arthropods. There is no information on effects on beneficial arthropods.

1.1.4 *Effects on experimental animals and* in vitro *test systems*

Trichlorfon is an insecticide that is moderately toxic for experimental animals. Oral LD_{50} values for technical trichlorfon in laboratory animals range from 400 to 800 mg/kg body weight and dermal LD_{50} values for the rat are greater than 2000 mg/kg body weight.

Trichlorfon poisoning causes the usual organophosphate cholinergic signs attributed to accumulation of acetylcholine at nerve endings.

Technical trichlorfon was shown to be moderately irritating to the eyes of rats, but was not irritating in skin tests on rabbits. Skin sensitization potential was demonstrated in guinea-pigs.

Short-term, oral toxicity studies were carried out on rats, dogs, monkeys, rabbits, and guinea-pigs. In a 16-week study on rats, a 4-year study on dogs, and a 26-week study on monkeys, no-observed-effect levels (NOELs) of 100 mg/kg diet, 50 mg/kg diet, and 0.2 mg/kg body weight (based on plasma, erythrocyte, or brain ChE activity) respectively, were determined. Inhalation exposure of rats, over 3 weeks, indicated a NOEL of 12.7 mg/m^3, based on the inhibition of plasma, erythrocyte, and brain ChE activity. Long-term toxicity/carcinogenicity studies were carried out on mice, rats, monkeys, and hamsters after oral, intraperitoneal, or dermal administration. An adverse effect on the gonads was seen following the oral exposure of mice and rats at dose levels of 30 mg/kg body weight and 400 mg/kg diet, respectively. In a 24-month study on rats and a 10-year study on monkeys, no-observed-adverse-effect levels (NOAELs) of 50 mg/kg diet and 0.2 mg/kg body weight, respectively, were determined. Available data do not provide evidence of carcinogenicity following the long-term exposure of test animals by several routes of administration.

Under physiological conditions, trichlorfon has been reported to have a DNA-alkylating property. The trichlorfon mutagenicity results have been both positive and negative. Dichlorvos may be responsible, either in part or in full, for the effects observed. Most of the *in vitro* mutagenicity studies on both bacterial and mammalian cells were positive while few of the *in vivo* studies produced a positive result.

Studies on mice, rats, and hamsters indicate that trichlorfon produces a teratogenic response in rats at doses high enough to produce maternal toxicity. Exposure of rats to 145 mg trichlorfon/kg diet, during gestation, caused fetal malformations. A gavage dose of 400 mg/kg body weight in hamsters also produced both maternal toxicity and a teratogenic response. The lowest dose by gavage that produced teratogenic effects in rats was 80 mg/kg body weight. The effects appear to be time specific in the gestation period. A NOEL of 8 mg/kg was determined in this gavage study.

NOELs of 8 mg/kg body weight and 200 mg/kg body weight were demonstrated for rats and hamsters, respectively. Teratogenic responses involving the central nervous system have also been reported for the pig and guinea-pig.

However, no teratogenic effects were observed in a 3-generation reproduction study on rats, in which high dose levels induced adverse reproductive effects. The NOEL in this study was 300 mg/kg diet.

Very high doses have produced neurotoxic effects in animals.

The active transformation product in mammals is dichlorvos, which is estimated to be at least 100 times more potent as an anticholinesterase than trichlorfon.

1.1.5 Effects on human beings

Several cases of acute poisoning from intentional (suicide) or accidental exposure have occurred. Signs and symptoms of intoxication were characteristic of AChE inhibition, such as exhaustion, weakness, confusion, excessive sweating and salivation, abdominal pains, vomiting, pinpoint pupils, and muscle spasms. In severe cases of poisoning, unconsciousness and convulsions developed and death usually resulted from respiratory failure. In cases where victims survived due to medical intervention, a delayed polyneuropathy, associated with weakness of the lower limbs, sometimes occurred a few weeks after exposure. In fatal cases, autopsy findings showed ischaemic changes in the brain, spinal cord, and vegetative ganglia, damage to the myelin sheath in the spinal cord and brain peduncles, and structural changes in the axons of peripheral nerves.

A few cases of occupational poisoning have occurred, mainly through the neglect of safety precautions. Occupational exposure at a work-place where air concentrations exceeded 0.5 mg/m^3 resulted in decreased plasma cholinesterase and changes in the EEG pattern. However, these were completely reversible on cessation of exposure. No cases of skin sensitization have been reported.

This compound has been extensively used for the treatment of schistosomiasis in humans. Administration of a single dose (7-12 mg/kg) resulted in cholinesterase inhibition in plasma and erythrocytes in the range of 40-60%, without cholinergic symptoms. However, mild symptoms were observed in cases with a repeated dose regimen. A high dose level (24 mg/kg) caused severe cholinergic symptoms.

1.2 Conclusions

- Trichlorfon is a moderately toxic organophosphorus ester insecticide. Over-exposure from handling during manufacture or use and accidental or intentional ingestion may cause serious poisoning.
- Trichlorfon exposure of the general population occurs mainly as a result of agricultural and veterinary practices, and in the treatment of *Schistosoma haematobium*.
- The reported trichlorfon intakes are far below the Acceptable Daily Intake established by FAO/WHO and should not constitute a health hazard for the general population.
- With good work practices, hygienic measures, and safety precautions, trichlorfon is unlikely to present a hazard for those occupationally exposed.

- Despite its high toxicity for non-target arthropods, trichlorfon has been used with few or no adverse effects on populations of organisms in the environment.

1.3 Recommendations

- For the health and welfare of workers and the general population, the handling and application of trichlorfon should only be entrusted to competently supervised and well-trained operators, who will follow adequate safety measures and apply trichlorfon according to good application practices.

- The manufacture, formulation, agricultural use, and disposal of trichlorfon should be carefully managed to minimize contamination of the environment, particularly surface waters.

- Regularly exposed worker and patient populations should undergo periodic health evaluations.

- Application rates of trichlorfon should be limited, to avoid effects on non-target arthropods. The insecticide should never be sprayed over water bodies or streams.

2. IDENTITY, PHYSICAL AND CHEMICAL PROPERTIES, ANALYTICAL METHODS

2.1 Identity

Trichlorfon was first prepared by Lorenz in 1952 and then by Barthel in 1954 by the reaction of dimethyl phosphite with chloral. It is a racemic mixture of dimethyl 2,2,2-trichloro-1-hydroxyethylphosphonate. Two molecules of trichlorfon are associated together (Lorenz et al., 1955).

Chemical structure:

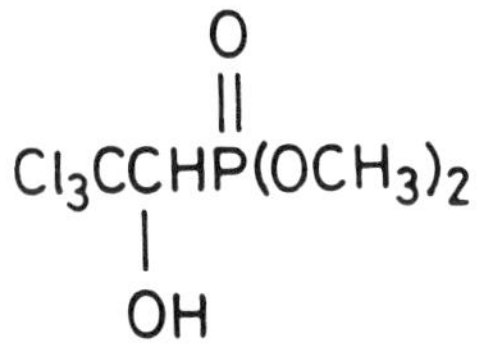

Chemical formula:	$C_4H_8Cl_3O_4P$
Relative molecular mass:	257.44
Common name:	trichlorfon (ISO)
Chemical name:	dimethyl 2,2,2-trichloro-1-hydroxyethylphosphonate
Synonyms:	chlorofos, DEP, DETF, dipterex, dimethyl 1-hydroxy- 2,2,2-trichloroethanephosphonate, *O,O*-dimethyl (2,2,2-trichloro-1-hydroxyethyl) phosphonate, metrifonate, foschlor, trichlorofon, trichlorphon

Trade names:	Agroforotox, Anthon, L 13/59, Bilarcil, Cekufon, Danex, Dipterex, Ditriphon, Dylox, Dyrex, Dyvon, Masoten, Metrifonate, Neguvon, Proxol, Tugon, Wotex
CAS registry number:	52-68-6
RTECS registry number:	TA 0700000
Impurities:	The purity of technical trichlofon was reported to be more than 98% (FAO/WHO, 1972). The main impurities are 2,2-dichlorovinyl dimethyl phosphate: dichlorvos (0-0.2%), trichloroacetaldehyde (0-0.05%), dichloroacetaldehyde (0-0.03%), methyl hydrogen 2,2,2-trichloro-1-hydroxyethylphosphonate; demethyl trichlorfon (0-0.3%), and water (less than 0.3%). The technical product also contains phosphoric acid, 2,2,2-trichloro-1-hydroxyethylphosphonic acid, and dimethyl phosphite (FAO/WHO, 1972; Melnikov et al., 1975).

2.2 Physical and chemical properties

Trichlorfon is a colourless crystalline powder that is stable at room temperature. It is slowly hydrolysed in acid media; the half-life is 526 days at pH 1-5 and 20 °C (Mühlmann & Schrader, 1957). Cleavage of one of the methyl ester groups takes place by acid hydrolysis. In alkaline media, however, trichlorfon is rapidly converted to dichlorvos and then hydrolytic products (see section 4.2).

Some physical properties are given in Table 1.

Table 1. Physical and chemical properties of trichlorfon[a]

Physical state	colourless crystals	
Melting point (°C)	83-84	
Boiling point (°C)	100 (0.1 mmHg)	
Vapour pressure (20 °C)	7.8×10^{-6} mmHg	
Volatility (20 °C)	0.022 mg/m^3	
Density	$^{20}_{4}$ 1.73	
Solubility in g/100 ml (25 °C)	water	15.4
	benzene	15.2
	chloroform	75.0
	diethyl ether	17.0
	n-hexane	0.08
Partition coefficient (octanol/water)	log P_{ow} 0.57	
Corrosiveness	corrosive to metals	

[a]From: Giang et al. (1954); FAO/WHO (1972); Dedek (1981); IARC (1983).

2.3 Conversion factors

1 ppm = 11.4 mg/m^3
1 mg/m^3 = 0.088 ppm, at 25 °C and 760 mmHg.

2.4 Analytical methods

There are several methods for the determination of trichlorfon, some of which are listed in Table 2. For formulation analysis, potentiometric titration of liberated chloride with standard silver nitrate ($AgNO_3$) has been recommended (Macdougall, 1964; Bennewitz & Foth, 1967). The total chlorine content is determined by refluxing with aqueous NaOH. On the other hand, treatment with ethanolamine at room temperature gives one molecule of hydrogen chloride from each molecule of trichlorfon. Polarography is also used (Giang & Caswell, 1957). However, extraction with ethyl acetate and gas-chromatographic determination are generally applied (Zweig & Sherma, 1972).

Table 2. Summary of analytical methods for the determination of trichlorfon

Sample medium	Sample preparation	Analytical conditions (Detector, column, column temperature	Detection limit	Recovery (%) (added level, mg/kg)	Comments	Reference
Formulation	refluxing with concentration NaOH	potentiometric titration with $AgNO_3$ of total Cl^-			determination of trichlorfon in formulations	MacDougall (1964)
	standing with ethanolamine for 1 h at room temperature	potentiometric titration of liberated HCl with $AgNO_3$			distinguishable between trichlorfon and dichlorvos	Bennewitz & Foth (1967)
	ethyl acetate ext.[a]	FTD-GC, 25% carbowax 20W, 1.5 m (5 ft) 195 °C, N_2, 120 ml/min	0.01 μg accuracy	± 1-2%	determination of trichlorfon in powder formulation	Zweig & Sherma (1972)
	dissolving in $CHCl_3$ and sililating with bis-(trimethylsilyl)-trifluoracetamide	FID-GC, 3% XE-60, 1.2 m, 110 °C, He 50 ml/min	relative standard deviation	1.3%	determination of trichlorfon in soluble powder formulation	Bowman & Dame (1974)

Table 2 (continued)

Formulation (continued)	acetylating with acetic anhydride-pyridine mixture (2:0.5) in CH_3CN	FTD-GC, 15% Apiezon L, 1 m, 160-200 °C, N_2, 60 ml/min	pg		determination of trichlorfon after acetylation	Vilceanu et al. (1973)
Residues in food	0.1 N H_2SO_4 diethyl ether	FTD-GC 16% XF-1150, 2 m (6 ft) 135 °C, He 25 ml/min	0.1 mg/kg	74-86 (0.1) 102-5 (12.5)	the extracts should be dialysed for 24 h before extraction	Zweig & Sherma (1972)
Crops, fish, chicken	$CH_3CN + H_2O/CHCH_3$ ext.[a] hexane - CH_3CN partition $CH_3CN: + H_2O$, evaporation, aq. layer/heptane washing NaCl, ether ext.[a]	FTD-GC, 20% carbowax 20 M, 1m, 150 °C, N_2 60 ml/min	5 µg/kg	90-100 (0.2) fat 72 (0.2)	some metabolites are also determined	Takase et al. (1972)
Crops, soil, animal tissues, water	$CHCl_3$ ext.; reext. with activated carbon/acetone (hexane sat.[a] NaCl ext. $CHCl_3$ + NaCl ext.; aq. phase/$CHCl_3$ ext. for animal tissue)	FPD-GC, 16% XF-1150, 2 m, 125 °C	2 µg/kg (water) 50 µg/kg (others)	100 (0.002-0.25) water, 94-104 (0.05-0.2) soil, 90-99 (0.05-50) plants, 82 (0.05-1.0) animal	determination of trichlorfon in forest environmental samples	Devine (1973)

Table 2 (continued)

Sample medium	Sample preparation	Analytical conditions (Detector, column, column temperature	Detection limit	Recovery (%) (added level, mg/kg)	Comments	Reference
Fruit	acetone ext.; 2% Na_2SO_4/hexane then ethyl acetate N_2 40 ml/min	FTD-or FPD-GC, 5% carbowax-20 M, 3 m, 160-180 °C	0.1 mg/kg	90-102% (1.0)	clean-up is not necessary for ethyl acetate extraction	Ferreira & Fernandes (1980)
Livestock products	CH_3CN ext.; 5% Na_2SO_4/$CHCl_3$ ext.[a] haxane-CH_3CN partition aq. CH_3CN/CH_2Cl_2 ext.[a]	FPD-GC, 3% Thermon 3000, 0.3 m, 120-170 °C, N_2 60 ml/min	2 μg/kg	90 (egg)-102 (milk) (0.4)	Salithion (same retention time) can be removed by washing with *n*-hexane	Imanaka et al. (1981)
Milk	$CHCl_3$ ext.	TLC, benzene-methyl acetate (3:1), enzymic determination after activation with ammonia	5 μg/kg	75-100 (0.02-0.4)	semi-quantitative determination separating dichlorvos	Fechner et al. (1971)
Feed	0.1% HCl ext.[a]; $CHCl_3$ reext.[a]	FPD-GC DB-1 (FSOT) 0.53 min x 30 m 120-150 °C (6 °C/min) He 10 ml/min	0.01 mg/kg	88 (50 ppm)	feed samples	Cox et al. (1989)

Table 2 (continued)

Crops	acetone or CH_3CN ext.; conc.[a] + NaCl reext.[a] with diethyl ether; Sep-pak C_{18} (silica gel) benzene/MeOH	FTD-GC, methyl silicon or phenyl-methyl silicon; (FSOT) 0.53 mm x 10 m, 160 °C	0.01 ng	70-99 (0.1 mg/kg)	sep-pak cartridge is very useful for simple clean-up	Ishizaka et al. (1986)
Serum	Serum + 0.1 mix well; M HCl (1 = 1) Sep-pak C_{18} (silica gel) 0.1 M HCl, 10% & 50% aq. MeOH	FTD-GC, CBP-1 (FSOT) 0.53 mm x 12 m 120 °C He 30 ml/min	2.5 ng/ml		extraction is not necessary for wide range of calibration curve (5 ~ 500 ng/ml)	Ameno et al. (1989)

[a] ext. = extraction.
reext. = reextraction.
sat. = saturated.
conc. = concentration.

Extraction with acetonitrile, reextraction with ether and gas-chromatographic determination with flame photometric detection (FPD) or flame thermionic detection (FTD) are standard procedures for the determination of residues. Trichlorfon is thermally decomposed during chromatography to give dimethyl phosphite which is then determined (Ferreira & Fernandes, 1980). Chloral generated by decomposition can be determined by electron-capture detector (Zweig & Sherma, 1972).

Acetylation or trimethylsilylation can stabilize trichlorfon for gas chromatography without decomposition (Vilceanu et al., 1973; Bowman & Dame, 1974). Trichlorfon itself has been successfully determined at a high sensitivity using a column, such as Thermon 3000 on Shimalite TPA. More recently, a GC- FTD method, based on on-column derivation by acetic anhydride, has been reported by Conrad et al. (1987). The response is linear over ranges of 0.1-2.0 ng. The method is applicable for the determination of trichlorfon in technical products and formulations, as well as for residues in crops and animal tissue samples.

The simultaneous detection (μg/kg) and identification of trichlorfon and other organophosphorus pesticides extracted from foods can be accomplished by using gas chromatography-mass spectrometry (Stan, 1977; Stan et al., 1977). Although the molecular ion cannot be measured by the electron impact (EI) ionization mass spectrum, an intense peak of the protonated molecular ion $(M+1)^+$ is observed in the chemical ionization (CI) mass spectrum. Thus, the latter is more sensitive and selective than the former in residue determination. Field desorption mass spectrum shows the protonated dimer ion $(2M+1)^+$ of trichlorfon besides the (M+1) ion (Schulten & Sun, 1981). The occurrence of such ions is helpful in confirming the identification of trichlorfon.

Thin-layer chromatography (TLC) is particularly useful for qualitative analysis. Systematic separation schemes for many organophosphorus pesticides have been proposed (Guth, 1967; Getz & Wheeler, 1968; Antoine & Mees, 1971; Ambrus et al., 1981). Levels of 0.1 μg trichlorfon can be detected using nitrobenzyl-pyridine reagent or silver nitrate and UV irradiation on silica gel or polyamide TLC. A TLC-enzyme inhibition technique that can be used for the determination of residues in organophosphorus pesticides was reviewed by Mendoza (1973). Trichlorfon itself is not a good inhibitor of cholinesterase (Winterlin et al., 1968), but treatment with ammonia on the plate, converting it into dichlorvos, is performed to enhance its sensitivity (Fechner et al., 1971).

Although high performance liquid chromatography (HPLC) has recently become an important technique in pesticide analysis, few data are available for trichlorfon (Szalontai, 1976; Daldrup et al., 1981, 1982).

Colorimetric methods have been applied for determining trichlorfon, based on the phosphomolybdate reaction (Sissons & Telling, 1970) and the Fujiwara reaction (Cerna, 1963; Giang et al., 1954).

A method to preconcentrate water samples for the measurement of trichlorfon was reported by Dedek et al. (1987).

The use of gas chromatographic detectors in HPLC has recently received increasing attention because of the growing need for high sensitivity and selectivity. The on-line combination of HPLC and these detectors, using a thermo spraying interface (TSP), has been applied successfully, because the advent of miniaturized HPLC systems has alleviated many of the difficulties including a loss of sensitivity associated with direct mobile phase introduction. In most cases, the techniques of HPLC separation, GC-FTD detection, and GC-MS confirmation can be successfully used in the analyses with TSP-HPLC-FTD and TSP-HPLC-MS (Gluckman et al., 1986).

The TSP-HPLC-FTD system has been successfully used to determine a polar and thermally unstable pesticide like trichlorfon in many samples, because high sensitivity and less matrix interference are achieved than with the HPLC-ultraviolet spectrophotometry (UV) system for pesticide residues. According to Gluckman's report (1986), trichlorfon can be detected at a level of 40 pg by TSP-HPLC-FTD and the residues in tomatoes and cabbage can be determined without any interference.

The characterization of several organophosphorus pesticides has been achieved using positive and negative ion "filament on" TSP-HPLC-MS. When ammonia gas is used as a reagent one, the base peak is $[M + NH_4]^+$ in the positive ion mode (PIM) for the organophosphorus pesticides examined, while the pesticides exhibited different fragmentation behaviour in the negative ion mode (NIM)

($[M]^-$ in the base peak). PIM shows a higher sensitivity for these compounds than NIM.

Trichlorfon and other organophosphorus pesticides can be detected at levels of 20-50 ng (minimum detection limit; s/n = 3) in the reconstructed ion chromatography of PIM-HPLC-MS. Since, a 100-fold to 1000-fold increase in sensitivity will be expected using single ion monitoring (SIM), the detection limits in PIM-TSP-HPLC-MS are rather similar to those in GC-NCI-MS and in direct liquid introduction (DLI)-HPLC-NCI-MS (Barcelo, 1987; Barcelo et al., 1988; Betowski & Jones, 1988).

The Joint FAO/WHO Codex Alimentarius Commission has given recommendations for the methods of analysis to be used in the determination of trichlorfon residues (FAO/WHO, 1989).

Because of the transformation of trichlorfon into dichlorvos, it is necessary to have a method for the simultaneous quantification of both of these compounds in biological studies. Such a method has been worked out by Nordgren (1981), and Nordgren et al. (1978, 1980, 1981), and has been correlated with the degree of enzyme inhibition. Similar methods have been used by Yakoub (1990).

3. SOURCES OF HUMAN AND ENVIRONMENTAL EXPOSURE

3.1 Natural occurrence

Trichlorfon is not a natural product. However, it is found as a metabolite of the insecticide butonate: butyric acid ester of trichlorfon (Dedek et al., 1979).

3.2 Industrial production

Trichlorfon was introduced as a commercial chemical in 1952. It is manufactured by reacting dimethyl phosphite with chloral (Barthel et al., 1954; Lorenz et al., 1955).

There is no record of the world production of trichlorfon. It is produced in Germany, Japan, and Spain and is believed to be produced also in Argentina, Brazil, China, Israel, Mexico, the Republic of Korea, and the USSR. The total production in western Europe was estimated to be about 2000 tonnes in 1977. The production in Japan has ranged from 613 to 1095 tonnes per year over the last decade (Japan Plant Protection Association, 1985, 1986, 1989).

3.3 Uses

Trichlorfon is a broad-spectrum insecticide that is particularly effective against *Diptera*. In agriculture, it is used mainly against insect pests in field and fruit crops. Trichlorfon is also used to control forest insects, in public health, and for the control of endo- and ectoparasites in/on domestic animals and fish.

Under the generic name of metrifonate, trichlorfon is used as an antihelminthic in humans and is one of the treatments of choice for infestation by *Schistosoma haematobium*, primarily in Africa (Snellen, 1981; Davis, 1986; Aden Abdi et al., 1987; Wilkins & Moore, 1987; Aden Abdi & Gustafsson, 1989; Yakoub, 1990; Aden Abdi, 1990). The usual regimen consists of three doses of 7.5 or 10 mg/kg, given at intervals of 14-21 days. Because of the lower costs in comparison with other treatments, metrifonate is particularly attractive for mass treatments. It has been given to millions of patients with schistosomiasis with only occasional mild side effects

(Nordgren, 1981). In order to obtain better patient compliance, Aden Abdi (1990) recently proposed a regimen of 3 x 5 mg, administered in one day (see section 9.2).

Metrifonate is also under consideration as a treatment for Alzheimer's disease (Hallak & Giacobini, 1989; Becker et al., 1990; Pomponi et al., 1990).

Table 3 gives an indication of the world-wide consumption of trichlorfon. Although the quantity is not reported, trichlorfon is used also in several other countries including Finland, Hungary, Malaysia, Mongolia, and the USSR. According to a Battelle report (1987), the total consumption of trichlorfon in 13 countries in 1987 was 851 tonnes as shown in Table 4, which also includes data from other sources.

The following formulations are used in agriculture: 50% emulsifiable concentrate, 95, 80, and 50% soluble powders, 50% wettable powders, 5 and 4% dusts, 5, 2.5, and 1% granules, 75, 50, 40, and 25% ultra-low volume concentrates. Some formulations mixed with other organophosphorus insecticides, such as malathion and ESP, or with carbamate insecticides, such as carbaryl, are also used.

The following formulations are used for animal treatments: 90, 80, and 50% soluble powders, 6% suspension, 11% solution, 50% injectable solution tablets. A 1% fly bait is also available, and a 0.1% preparation against house-ants. For antihelminthic preparations, trichlorfon can be used in combination with atropine, fenbendazole, or thiabendazole.

Tablets containing 100 mg active ingredient metrifonate are used in the treatment of schistosomiasis in humans.

Table 3. World usage of trichlorfon

Year	Usage (tonne)	References
1980	3159	Battelle (1982)
1983	2349	Battelle (1984)
1987	851	Battelle (1987)

Table 4. Usage of trichlorfon[a]

Country	Usage (tonne)	Year	Main use
France	-	1987	
Italy	10.2	1987	vines
Turkey	16.4	1987	vegetables
FRG[b]	19.9	1984	sugar beet
United Kingdom[b]	0.8	1984	sugar beet
Spain	155.3	1987	vines, vegetables, olives
Czechoslovakia[c]	-	1983	
Sweden[c]	5.7	1982	agriculture, hygiene
Japan	279.7	1987	potatoes, other vegetables
Korea, Republic	79.0		forests, apples
India	-		
Indonesia	6.0	1987	soybeans
Thailand[c]	19.0	1978	
Philippines[b]	-	1984	
USA	454.0[d]	1978	field crops, alfalfa, forests, cotton, vegetables
	1.8	1987	alfalfa
Mexico	133.1	1987	maize, cotton, tobacco, tomatoes, sugar cane, soybeans
Brazil	145.3		soybeans, cotton, wheat
Egypt	-		
South Africa	24.6		maize
Kenya[c]	-	1983	

[a] From: Battelle (1987).
[b] From: Battelle (1984).
[c] Information through IRPTC (International Register of Potentially Toxic Chemicals).
[d] From: IARC (1983).

4. ENVIRONMENTAL TRANSPORT, DISTRIBUTION, AND TRANSFORMATION

Following aerial application, trichlorfon is distributed to the air, soil, water, trees, plants, and other media. With rainfall, trichlorfon penetrates into the lower soil layers and moves into the aquatic environment.

4.1 Transport and distribution

4.1.1 Air

The air/water partition coefficient of trichlorfon was determined to be $< 5.0 \times 10^{-7}$, indicating that the distributed amount in air is much smaller than that in water and is, in fact, negligible (Kawamoto & Urano, 1989).

4.1.2 Water

One and two days after the aerial application of trichlorfon to a forest at the rate of 1.0 kg/ha, a small amount of the compound was found in creek water (Pieper & Richmond, 1976). Trichlorfon was also detected in water samples in sprayed forests in Canada (Sergeant & Zitko, 1979).

Rainfall caused run-off of trichlorfon from the sprayed steppe zone into ponds (IRPTC/GKNT, 1983). In an agricultural region of the USSR, trichlorfon migrated into drainage water and was transferred across a significant distance, depending on the rainfall (Zakharov, 1980).

4.1.3 Soil

Because of its high water-solubility (15.4 g/100 ml), there was some downward movement of trichlorfon through soil with water. When sprayed twice on an apple orchard, the insecticide was detected in soil layers of 0-10 cm and 10-20 cm depth, 10 days after the last treatment (Naishtein et al., 1973).

Trichlorfon applied to the soil surface at the rate of 2.4 kg a.i./ha did not move significantly into the lower layers by leaching (Baida, 1970); when applied at a high rate of 60 kg/ha, the compound penetrated into the 60-cm layer of the soil (Naishtein, 1976).

It has been shown, in different soils, that the disappearance of the insecticide (initial concentration; 10 mg/kg) is very rapid during the first few days following application and considerably slower thereafter. The levels of trichlorfon residues in a soil without plants were 5.2, 2.1, and 0.9 mg/kg on the 5th, 11th, and 21st days after application, respectively. However, in soils with tomato, cabbage, and potato plants, trichlorfon levels decreased more rapidly to 2.1, 1.0, and 0.6 mg/kg, respectively, on the 5th day, 0.7, 0.5, and 0.3 mg/kg on the 11th day, and 0.6, 0.3, and 0.2 mg/kg on the 21st day after treatment. Only a small amount of trichlorfon was detected after 30 days. The rate of disappearance in soils was dependent on the vegetation (Ivanova & Molozhanova, 1974).

4.2 Abiotic degradation

The proposed degradation pathways of trichlorfon in the environment are shown in Fig. 1.

In alkaline buffers and seawater (pH 8.1), trichlorfon is rearranged via dehydrochlorination to yield the more potent cholinesterase inhibitor, dichlorvos; however, in acidic buffers or in fresh water (pH 5.3), it is stable. At more alkaline pH values, the anticholinesterase activity disappears slowly (Ecobichon, 1979). At pH 5.5 and above, degradation to dichlorvos occurs at detectable rates (Dedek, 1981).

On photolysis in water under ultraviolet radiation (UVR), trichlorfon was rapidly converted to dichlorvos (2) and two unidentified products. These two products decomposed further on prolonged irradiation. Photodegradation appears to be much slower in the solid state than in aqueous solution (Giovanoli-Jakubczak et al., 1971).

[^{32}P]-trichlorfon on glass plates was photodecomposed by 7% after a 5-h exposure to UVR (500 W, 200-600 nm) and by 6% after a 20-h exposure to sunlight. A trace amount of dimethyl hydrogen phosphate (5) (see Fig. 1) and methyl hydrogen phosphate (7) were identified as photodegradation-products, whereas dichlorvos (2) was not detected among the photodegradation-products on the glass plates in either case (Dedek et al., 1979).

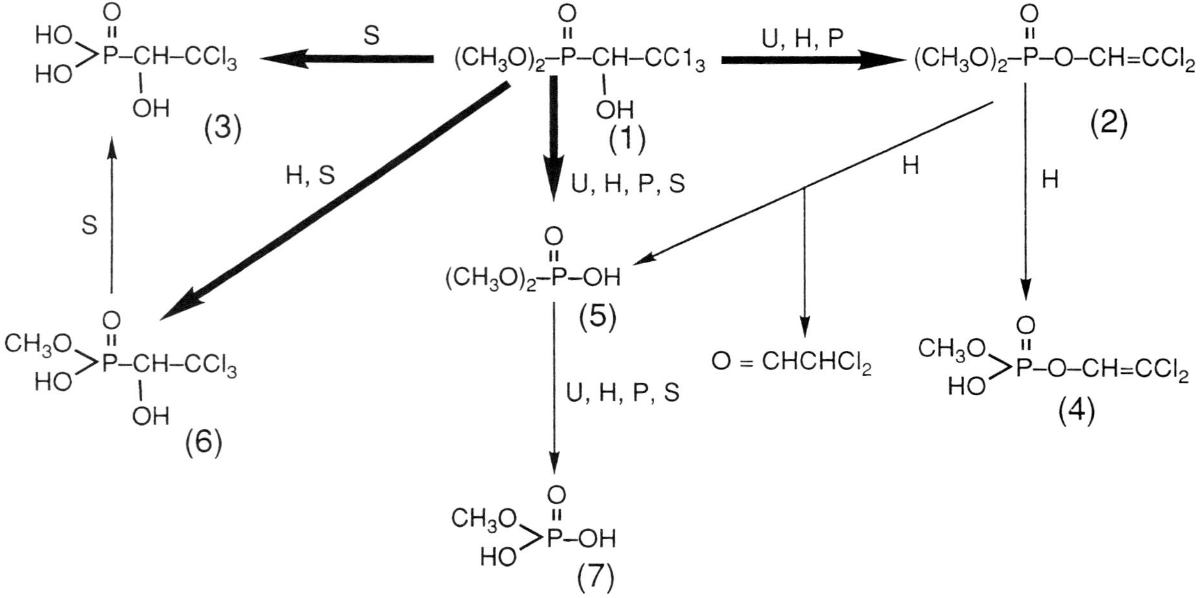

Fig 1. Proposed degradation pathways of trichlorfon in the environment. Photolysis (U); Hydrolysis (H); Soil and microorganisms (S); Plants (P).

WHO 91702

Trichlorfon is fairly stable in acidic solutions, but unstable in neutral and basic solutions. The half-life of chloroform-extractable radioactivity in buffer solutions at 40 °C is 46.4 days at pH 2, 16 days at pH 5, 3.75 days at pH 6, 19 h at pH 7, 8.8 h at pH 8, and 75 min at pH 10. Dichlorvos (2), the demethylated derivative of trichlorfon (6), dimethyl hydrogen phosphate (5) and methyl hydrogen phosphate (7) were identified as degradation products, but they were not quantified (see Fig. 1; Dedek et al., 1979).

In other studies, the half-life of trichlorfon at 100 mg/litre in sterilized water-ethanol (99:1) phosphate buffers at 25 ± 3 °C, was reported to be more than 1000 weeks at pH 4.5, 3.5 weeks at pH 6.0, 0.4 weeks at pH 7.0, and 0.13 weeks at pH 8.0. It was concluded that the disappearance was mainly due to the conversion of trichlorfon to dichlorvos via dehydrochlorination (Chapman & Cole, 1982). In another study, the half-lives for the formation of dichlorvos from trichlorfon at pH 7, pH 7.5, and pH 8 were reported by Hofer (1981) to be 27, 9, and 3 h, respectively.

Formulated trichlorfon was applied to sterilized and non-sterilized soils with a 60% moisture content, and incubated at ambient temperature under natural sunlight. At concentrations of both 13 and 132 mg/kg, the levels of insecticide decreased to less than the detection limit within 40 and 50 days, respectively, under both sterilized and non-sterilized conditions. It appears that the insecticide is readily subjected to abiotic degradation in soil (Yurovskaya & Zhulinskaya, 1974).

4.3 Biodegradation

The metabolic fate of [^{14}C]-trichlorfon labelled at the methoxy group has been studied in culture media of nodule-forming bacteria, such as *Rhizobium leguminosarum* and *Rhizobium trifolii*. After incubation for 10 days at 30 °C, the unchanged parent compound (19-25%) together with dimethyl hydrogen phosphate (18- 25%) (5) and methyl hydrogen phosphate (0.6-1%) (7) was recovered from the media. In addition, a trace amount of [^{14}C] carbon dioxide was evolved during the same period (Salama et al., 1975) (see Fig. 1).

In contrast, a demethylated derivative (6) of trichlorfon and 2,2,2- trichlorohydroxyethylphosphonic acid (3) were shown to be the major metabolites in the culture media of *Aspergillus niger*, *Penicillium notatum*, and *Fusarium* spp. (Zayed et al., 1965).

4.4 Environmental fate

The metabolism of [^{14}C]-trichlorfon labelled at the methoxy group has been studied in plants of the broad bean (*Vicia faba*) and clover (*Trifolium alexandrinum*). The roots of the plants were immersed in a phosphate buffer at pH 6 containing [^{14}C]-trichlorfon at a concentration of 50 mg/litre, and grown for 5 or 10 days in the greenhouse. At harvest, the buffer solution as well as the roots of the two plants contained unchanged parent compound and dimethyl hydrogen phosphate (5) together with a trace amount of methyl hydrogen phosphate (7) (Salama et al., 1975) (see Fig. 1).

Following the application of [^{32}P]-trichlorfon to stems or leaves, the insecticide disappeared from tomato, potato, and cotton plants with half-lives of 20-57 h in the greenhouse, and from plums, apples, cherries, peas, and wheat plants with half-lives of 0.5-7.5 days in the field. Characterization of metabolites was not possible because of their volatility (Dedek et al., 1979).

When formulated trichlorfon (0.2%) was sprayed on cabbage and onion plants at a rate of 1200 litre/ha, rapid conversion to dichlorvos occurred. One day after treatment, the treated leaves of cabbage and onion plants contained the highest residues of dichlorvos (0.09-0.51 mg/kg) together with the parent compound (0.79-3.1 mg/kg). Trichlorfon disappeared from the leaves with a half-life of less than 3 days, and dichlorvos decreased to less than the detection limit within 15 days (Baida, 1975).

5. ENVIRONMENTAL LEVELS AND HUMAN EXPOSURE

5.1 Environmental levels

5.1.1 Air

When 2% trichlorfon was applied at a rate of 30 ml/m^2, its vapour was detected in the air. The initial concentration of 0.1 mg/m^3 decreased rapidly to 0.05-0.01 mg/m^3 within 2-3 days. Trichlorfon was not detected after 30 days (Degtyareva et al., 1977). After handspraying in a vineyard at 2 and 6 kg/ha, air concentrations of 0.0003 and 0.001 mg/m^3, respectively, were measured. Average daily concentrations of trichlorfon and its maximum single concentration in the Ukrainian Republic were 0.0003 and 0.0004 mg/m^3, respectively (IRPTC/GKNT, 1983).

5.1.2 Water

When an 18% aqueous solution of trichlorfon was sprayed on a forest at a rate of approximately 1 kg/ha from a helicopter, the residues were 23.4-51.9 and 8.7-12.1 μg/litre in the creek water on the first and second day after application, respectively (Pieper & Richmond, 1976).

According to the monitoring programmes in Canada in 1976 and 1977, water samples in the forests where trichlorfon was sprayed were contaminated with 0.062-1.0 μg/litre of the insecticide in most of the year's samples in 1976, but the concentration in samples in 1977 were considerably lower, with a maximum value of 0.058 μg/litre (Sergeant & Zitko, 1979).

Trichlorfon was measured in soil water at 0.001 (1970), 0.02 (1971), and 0.001 mg/litre (1972) on average 1.5-2 months after application (IRPTC/GKNT, 1983).

When trichlorfon was sprayed over a mixed boreal forest in New Brunswick (Canada) at a rate of 1.14 kg/ha, concentrations in stream water were approximately 95 μg/litre initially and below detection limit (0.05 μg/litre) two weeks after treatment (Sundaram & Varty, 1989).

5.1.3 Soil

Trichlorfon was one of the chemicals found at hazardous waste sites in the USA (Kokoszka & Flood, 1989). Levels were not specified.

After the spraying of a vineyard at 2 or 6 kg/ha, trichlorfon levels measured in the soil were 0.24 and 0.48 mg/kg, respectively, on the day of treatment. One day later, the levels in the soil were 0.49 and 1.03 mg/kg, and 15 days later, 0.002 and 0.02 mg/kg. The average level of trichlorfon in the soil in the Kherson Region was 0.01 mg/kg (1970), 0.17 mg/kg (1971) and 0.002 mg/kg (1972). After spraying a forest at 0.8 kg/ha over a 200-ha area (160 kg total), monitoring soil over the area gave estimates of 29.9 kg trichlorfon remaining in the soil, 5 days after application and 0.43 and 0.25 kg after 10 and 14 days, respectively. All the trichlorfon measured was in the top 10 cm of soil. No trichlorfon was found 18 days after spraying (IRPTC/GKNT, 1983).

After aerial spraying of trichlorfon over a mixed boreal forest in New Brunswick (Canada) at a rate of 1.14 kg/ha, residues in soil dissipated from 3 mg/kg initially to levels below the detection limit (0.05 mg/kg) in about two weeks (Sundaram & Varty, 1989).

5.1.4 Residues in plants and animals

An 18% aqueous solution of trichlorfon was applied by helicopter at 6.1 litre/ha to a forest. The residues on days 1, 2, 8, and 15 after aerial treatment were 11.2-12.6 mg/kg, 3.8-10.4 mg/kg, 0.8-1.6 mg/kg and below detection limit-0.6 mg/kg, respectively, on Douglas fir, 68.2-81.7 mg/kg, 40.3-59.4 mg/kg, 3.9-4.5 mg/kg and below detection limit, respectively, on willow, and 43.1-113.0 mg/kg, 4.3-30.0 mg/kg, 5.3-6.3 mg/kg, and below the detection limit-2.1 mg/kg, respectively, on grasses (detection limit: 0.1 mg/kg) (Pieper & Richmond, 1976).

Trichlorfon was detected in all song birds caught in the area (60.7 ha), 76 h after spraying at the rate of 1.1 kg/ha. The residues of trichlorfon were found at 0.01 mg/kg for blue jays and crested fly-catchers and at 0.013-0.04 mg/kg for baltimore oriols (Kurtz & Studholme, 1974).

When trichlorfon was sprayed at a rate of 1.14 kg a.i./ha over a mixed boreal forest in New Brunswick (Canada), the initial residues in foliage ranged from 10.8 to 17.3 mg/kg fresh weight, but dissipated rapidly to 2.6 to 6.5 mg/kg in three days (Sundaram & Varty, 1989).

5.2 Residues in food

5.2.1 Crops

The results of supervised trials involving foliar treatment of various crops with trichlorfon are summarized in Table 5.

Leafy vegetables, such as lettuce, spinach, and Chinese raddish leaves showed high residues of trichlorfon (several mg/kg or more) shortly after application. The trichlorfon residues in Chinese raddish leaves were about ten times higher than those in the roots. Among fruits, strawberries, raspberries, black currants, and red currants were found to contain higher trichlorfon residues than other fruits, such as citrus. The results in Table 5 showed that the residues decreased rapidly with time after application.

During the period 1987-88, 764 home-grown and imported wheat samples were analysed for pesticide residues in the United Kingdom. Trichlorfon was not found at, or above, the reporting limit of 0.1 mg/kg (Osborne et al., 1989).

Following normal field application (in a field trial) of trichlorfon in Portugal to Portuguese cabbage and broccoli, residue levels decreased to below the MRL of 0.5 mg/kg in 10 days for the Portuguese cabbage and two weeks for the broccoli. The difference in time is mainly ascribed to the much larger surface area exposed in the case of the broccoli (Magalhaes et al., 1989).

The surveillance of trichlorfon residues on over twenty crops in Hungary revealed that about 90.1% of the samples contained residues at levels below 0.02 mg/kg (Anon. 1978a).

Trichlorfon residues on spinach and lettuce after spraying were somewhat higher in green-house crops than in field crops in West Germany (Stobwasser & Kirchhoff, 1968).

Table 5. Residues of trichlorfon in crops

Crop/ Country	Application (spray)			Residues (mg/kg) on the day of spraying or at intervals [days] after application[a]								Reference
				Day								
	no.	kg/ha	formulation[b]	0	1/3	4/6	7/9	10/12	13/15	17/19	21	
Cabbage												
Finland		ns				0.6			0.5	0.4 [18-21]	0.2 [27-29]	Anon.(1978b)
Japan	6	2-5	EC-50			0.14-0.05	0.08-0.03					FAO/WHO (1979)
	8	2-5				0.23-0.07	0.05-0.03					
USSR	4	2.0	EC		0.79-0.27	0.17		0.09	0.07		0.007 [30]	Baida (1975)
Chinese cabbage												
Japan	3	2.0	EC-50						0.13-0.04	0.09-0.02 [18-21]		Hiramatsu & Furutani (1977)
	5	2.0						0.06	0.05			FAO/WHO (1979)
	6	2.0						0.13	0.09			
	1	0.75			0.19-0.12		0.05		0.03			

Table 5 (continued)

Lettuce											
Finland	1	1.2	WP-80	34-26	5.6	0.75	0.25	0.13		0.01	Abbasov (1972)
USA	1	0.6	WP-50	1.6	0.8	0.3	0.7		0.3	0.2	FAO/WHO (1976)
	1	1.2		0.8	0.8	0.6	nd		0.3		
	1	0.6			1.2		0.3		0.3	nd	
	5	1.2						0.5			
	6	1.2							nd		
	7	1.2						0.2			
Head lettuce											
Finland	1	1.2	WP-50	22.8		1.5	0.31		0.04	0.01	FAO/WHO (1976)
	1	1.2		31.2		1.1	0.17		0.06	nd	
FRG	1	0.75	EC-50	8.1	1.8	0.54	0.41	0.20	nd	nd	FAO/WHO (1976)
	1	0.75		15.9	4.6	0.21	0.08	0.14	0.05	nd	
	1	0.45		5.8	1.8	0.22	0.09	nd	nd	nd	
	1	0.45		4.8	4.3	0.27	nd	nd	nd	nd	
Leaf lettuce											
Finland	1	1.2	WP-80	33.5		2.6	0.61			0.03	FAO/WHO (1976)
	1	1.2		26.4		1.3	0.23			0.02	

Table 5 (continued)

Crop/ Country	Application (spray)			Residues (mg/kg) on the day of spraying or at intervals [days] after application[a]								Reference
				Day								
	no.	kg/ha	formul-ation[b]	0	1/3	4/6	7/9	10/12	13/15	17/19	21	
USA	2	1.2	WP-50		6.3	1.3	nd		nd			FAO/WHO (1976)
	2	1.2			3.5	1.1	nd		nd			
	2	1.2			3.8-0.8	0.8-0.1	0.4-nd					
	2	1.2			97.6	9.2	6.0		3.9			
Red cabbage												
Netherlands	1	1.0	WP-80				0.05-0.03					Anon.(1978c)
Savoy cabbage												
Netherlands	1	1.0	WP-50				0.36-0.12					Anon.(1978c)
Parsley												
Hungary	1	0.8	WP-50		0.2	0.02	0.01/0.01					FAO/WHO (1976)

Table 5 (continued)

Brussel sprouts								
Netherlands	3	1.2	WP-80	0.4- 0.15	0.4- 0.15		0.13- 0.08	Anon. (1978c)
	4	1.2		0.9- 0.08	0.1- 0.08		0.05- 0.03	
Kale								
Netherlands	1	1.0	WP-80				0.33- 0.12	Anon. (1978c)
Kohlrabi								
Netherlands	1	1.0	WP-80				0.02- 0.01	Anon. (1978c)
Spinach								
Netherlands	1	1.0	WP-80			5.3- 3.4		FAO/WHO (1976)
	1	1.0				6.2- 2.1		

Table 5 (continued)

Crop/ Country	Application (spray)			Residues (mg/kg) on the day of spraying or at intervals [days] after application[a]								Reference
				Day								
	no.	kg/ha	formulation[b]	0	1/3	4/6	7/9	10/12	13/15	17/19	21	
Spinach (greenhouse)												
Netherlands	1	1.1	WP-50	33.3-23.3	5.5-2.9	3.4-1.2	1.3-0.4	0.9-0.2	0.4-0.2	0.5-0.1		FAO/WHO (1976)
	1	1.1		4.5-1.9	3.1-1.2	0.8-0.4	0.5-0.25	0.3-0.2	0.1-0.06			
Spinach (under frame)												
FRG	1	0.75	WP-50		4.4			2.4			1.6	FAO/WHO (1976)
	1	0.75		30	21.5	5.2	1.2	2.2			0.25	
Spinach (outdoor)												
Canada	2	1.1	WP			0.6	0.2		nd			FAO/WHO (1976)
	2	1.1				39	3.5		nd			
FRG	1	0.75				2.0	1.6	0.7	0.35			FAO/WHO (1976)
	1	0.75				0.4	0.02					
	1	ca. 1.5	WP-80			19.8	1.8					
	1	0.75	WP-50	34	6.0	0.85	0.15	0.15				
	1	0.75	WP-50	30		1.7	0.3	0.08				
	1	0.75		30	13.2	5.6	1.0	1.0				

Table 5 (continued)

Netherlands	1	0.5	WP-50	6.5-5.7	2.7-1.2	2.1- 0.08	0.6-0.1	0.3-0.2				FAO/WHO (1976)
	1	0.63		2.2-1.8	1.1-0.4	0.6-nd	0.2-0.1	0.2-nd				
	1	1.9		1.4-0.5		0.3- 0.05	0.01-nd					
	1	0.7		1.4-0.6	0.3-0.2	0.4-nd	0.7-nd					
USA	2	1.1				11.2	0.3		0.3			FAO/WHO (1976)
	2	1.1					0.9		0.4			
	2	1.1				1.8	0.2		nd			
Lima bean												
USA	1	2.22	EC								0.07- 0.02 [44]	FAO/WHO (1976)
Chinese radish												
Japan												
(leaf)	5	2.0	EC-50		2.76- 0.22	0.26- 0.09	0.07- 0.02					FAO/WHO (1979)
(root)	5	2.0			0.12- 0.07	0.07- 0.03	0.05- 0.01					
(leaf)	8	2.0			1.4- 0.9	0.77- 0.1	0.09- 0.03					

Table 5 (continued)

Crop/ Country	Application (spray)			Residues (mg/kg) on the day of spraying or at intervals [days] after application[a]								Reference
				Day								
	no.	kg/ha	formulation[b]	0	1/3	4/6	7/9	10/12	13/15	17/19	21	
Chinese radish												
Japan												
(root)	8	2.0			0.12-0.08	0.04-0.03	0.04-0.01					FAO/WHO (1979)
(leaf)	8	1.5-2.0	not stated		1.4-0.22	0.77-0.10	0.09-0.03					
Onion												
USSR	4	2.0	EC		2.7-3.1	0.90-1.2	0.02-0.77		nd-0.04		nd [30]	Baida (1975)
Potato												
Japan	6	2.0	EC-50				0.03-0.02	0.02-nd				FAO/WHO (1979)
Egg plant												
Japan	5	1.0	EC-50			0.03-0.02	0.01-nd	nd				FAO/WHO (1979)
	8	1.0				0.02	0.007-nd					

Table 5 (continued)

Green pepper											
Hungary	1	1.0	WP-50	0.13	0.06	0.05	0.03	0.02	0.02 [16]		Anon. (1978a)
Tomato (glasshouse)											
Netherlands	1	1.2	WP-50		0.03-nd						FAO/WHO (1976)
	1	1.2			0.13-nd						Abbasov (1972)
Apple											
Netherlands	1	1.2	WP					0.9-0.6			Anon. (1978c)
	1	1.2						1.9-0.1			Anon. (1978c)
Grape											
Japan **(unsacked)**	1-5	1.0	EC-50	1.6-0.8	1.4-0.28	0.9-0.4	0.4-0.26		0.15-0.1		Hiramatsu & Furutani (1978)
(sacked)				0.15	0.07	0.08	0.06		0.06		
Lemon											
USA	1	4.5	WP-80							nd[52-59]	Iwata et al. (1979)
Orange											
USA	1	4.5	WP-80							nd [52-59]	Iwata et al. (1979)

Table 5 (continued)

Crop/ Country	Application (spray)			Residues (mg/kg) on the day of spraying or at intervals [days] after application[a]								Reference
				Day								
	no.	kg/ha	formulation[b]	0	1/3	4/6	7/9	10/12	13/15	17/19	21	
Mandarin orange												
Japan	5	3.0	EC-50								nd [27-29]	FAO/WHO (1979)
Kaki persimmon												
Japan	3	3g/ tree	EC-50		0.57-0.53	0.36			0.3-0.25			FAO/WHO (1979)
Raspberry												
Finland	2	0.8g/ linear	not stated						5.6			Anon. (1978b)
		0.5-0.6g/ plant								2.9-0.7 [18-21]		Anon. (1978b)
Strawberry												
Japan	3	2.0	EC-50						1.4	0.31 [18-21]		FAO/WHO (1979)
	5	2.0				4.6			0.75			
	3	3.0							2.12	0.46 [18-21]		
	5	3.0					3.31		1.06			

Table 5 (continued)

Strawberry												
Japan (continued)	1	1.6-2.4								0.02 [18-21]		
	3	2-3	not stated					2.1-1.4		0.46-0.33 [20-21]		
	5	2-3	not stated			4.6-3.3		1.1-0.74				
Water melon												
not stated	6	2.0	EC-50				0.008					FAO/WHO (1979)
Black currant												
Finland		1.3g/ plant	not stated						2.6		0.2 [27-29]	Anon.(1978b)
Red currant												
Finland		1.6g/ plant	not stated						25		12 [27-29]	Anon.(1978b)
Rye-grass												
USA	1	1.1	5% bait	37.5		3.1	1.9				0.1	van Middelem et al. (1972)
Cotton												
USA	4	3.7-1.4	WP-50		79	4						Isaac et al. (1965)

Table 5 (continued)

Crop/ Country	Application (spray)			Residues (mg/kg) on the day of spraying or at intervals [days] after application[a]								Reference
				Day								
	no.	kg/ha	formulation[b]	0	1/3	4/6	7/9	10/12	13/15	17/19	21	
Sugar beet												
Japan	6	1.5	EC-50				0.05-0.02		0.04-0.02			FAO/WHO (1979)
	8	1.5					0.04-0.02		0.024-0.020			
Finland	2	0.64	not stated								0.05 [48]	Anon. (1978b)
	6	1.5	not stated			0.24-0.06			0.07-0.02			
	8	1.5	not stated			0.26-0.05			0.08-0.02			

[a] nd = not detectable;
ns = not stated.

[b] WP = Wettable powder;
EC = Emulsifiable concentrate.

No trichlorfon residues were found in a survey of pesticide residues on crops (total samples: 697) collected from a Tokyo market from April 1984 to March 1989 (detection limit: 0.005 mg/kg) (Nagayama et al., 1986, 1987, 1988, 1989).

Cucumber vines were sprayed to run-off with 0.05% trichlorfon aqueous solution, and the fruits sampled over a period of time. The half-life of trichlorfon was 1.76 days (Hameed et al., 1980).

Grape products were prepared in a laboratory from grapes harvested 1 day after the last application of trichlorfon. Trichlorfon residues were detected at levels of 140%, 120%, 159%, and 0.4% of the originally applied concentration in the grape juice, raisins, wines, and brandies, respectively, and the dichlorvos concentrations in the wines were higher than those in the grapes from which the wines were made (Hiramatsu & Furutani, 1978).

Residues of 0.0002-0.006 mg trichlorfon and dichlorvos/kg were detected in 8 out of 40 flower honeys in Bulgaria (Tsvetkova et al., 1981).

5.2.2 *Milk*

The results of supervised trials in which cows were treated with trichlorfon via several routes of exposure and the residues in the milk measured are summarized in Table 6.

Trichlorfon residues in cow's milk were mainly studied in animals that were administered the pesticide orally. The reports showed relatively high levels and a gradual disappearance of trichlorfon in the milk of treated cows. The residue values in FAO/WHO report (1979) were much higher than those in others (Table 6).

To control botflies, a 11.2% aqueous solution of trichlorfon was applied dermally to lactating cows. Maximum residues of trichlorfon and dichlorvos were found in the first milking (0.2 and 0.03 mg/litre, respectively) and were still detectable in the third milking. Storage and short-term heating of the milk did not essentially degrade the insecticide, but, with boiling, an accelerated transformation of trichlorfon to dichlorvos took place (Fechner et al., 1968).

Table 6. Residues of trichlorfon in milk of cows after application

Method of application	Residues (mg/kg) in milk after application															Reference
	mg/kg	1 h	2 h	3 h	4 h	6 h	8 h	9 h	10 h	12 h	20 h	24 h	32-72 h	96 h	168 h	
Dermal	80		0.1-0.25				0.05-0.25						0.05			Mollhoff (1971)
Dermal	36						0.1-0.2					0.05				Mollhoff (1971)
Dermal	100						0.1-0.2				0.05-0.1		0.01			Mollhoff (1971)
Dermal	100									0.05-0.1		0.05				Mollhoff (1971)
Oral	3	0.033		0.091		0.080		0.052				0.003	0.001			Nakahara et al. (1972)
Oral	30	0.56		0.33		0.25		0.16				0.007	0.001			Nakahara et al. (1972)
Oral	1[a]	0.034		0.029				0.021				0.009	0.001			Nakahara et al. (1972)

Table 6. (continued)

Intramuscular[b]	25	2.4	1.3	0.7	0.5	0.25	0.1			Dedek & Schwarz (1966)
Pour-on[d]	20	1.2	0.5	0.3	0.2	0.1	0.05			FAO/WHO[c] (1979)
Pour-on[e]	20	0.2	0.3	0.35	0.35	0.2	0.1			FAO/WHO[c] (1979)
Pour-on[f]	30					0.45		0.05	0.01	Dedek & Schwarz (1966)

[a] 1 mg trichlorfon/kg body weight for 5 days.
[b] 50% trichlorfon in polyethylene glycol.
[c] Data cited to fit in this table.
[d] 2% trichlorfon in mineral oil.
[e] 2% trichlorfon in vegetable oil.
[f] 5.7% in aqueous solution.

Treatment of cows with 0.25 or 0.5% aqueous solution of trichlorfon resulted in residues in milk of 0.02 and 0.7 mg/litre, respectively, within the first 72 h following treatment. The levels of trichlorfon were higher in the morning than in the evening flow (IRPTC/GKNT, 1983).

The trichlorfon residues in cow's milk were in direct proportion to the veterinary use of the insecticide on the cows. Heat processing of milk had little effect on trichlorfon residues. However, evaporation or spray drying of the milk reduced the residue levels considerably (Konrad et al., 1975).

5.2.3 Meat

Trichlorfon residues in pigs and sheep treated with the chemical under supervised trial conditions are shown in Table 7. The results revealed that trichlorfon residues in pork rapidly disappear; they were below the detection limit (0.01 mg/kg) 24 h after subcutaneous application of 25 mg/kg body weight. The residues following spray treatment of sheep against harmful insects decreased to below the detection limit (0.01 mg/kg) after 168 h (Dedek & Schwarz, 1970a).

^{32}P-labelled trichlorfon was poured evenly on to 600 cm^2 areas of the freshly shorn backs of sheep at a rate of 20 mg/kg. Only a minimal concentration (0.1 mg/kg) of the insecticide was detected in the blood of the sheep. However, trichlorfon levels in the blood of cattle were higher than those in the blood of sheep at a similar dose. When special solvents were used for the preparation of the trichlorfon solution and the dose was increased to 50 mg/kg, the level of residues in the blood of the sheep increased to 1.2 mg/litre (Dedek & Schwarz, 1970b).

Six USSR reports were available concerning supervised trials on pigs (7 mg/kg in meat and 12 mg/kg in fat after unspecified treatment; Yonova & Zhecheva, 1974), and sheep (Nepoklonov & Bukshtynov, 1971). According to the English summaries of the reports, the trichlorfon was rapidly absorbed and distributed among various organs and tissues, then metabolized and eliminated.

Table 7. Residues of trichlorfon in various meats after experimental application

Animal	Method of application	mg/kg or g/m^3	Residues (mg/kg) after application												Reference
			1 h	2 h	3 h	4 h	6 h	12 h	24 h	48 h	72 h	120 h	168 h	240 h	
Hen	spray	150 g/m^3					1.26		0.96	ND					Dmitriyev (1970)
Pig	subcu-taneous	25 mg/kg	6	5	3-4	2-3	1	0.1	0.01						Dedek & Schwarz (1970a)
Sheep	spray	4 g/m^3							2.3		0.8	0.6	trace	ND[a]	Nepoklonov & Bukshtynov (1971)

[a] ND = not detectable.

5.2.4 *Poultry and eggs*

The trichlorfon contents of the organs of hens treated externally with 1-8% aqueous solutions were 0.03-1.5 mg/kg, 0.01-0.7 mg/kg, 0.04-1.0 mg/kg, 0.02-0.8 mg/kg, 0.01-1.5 mg/kg or 0.02-0.9 mg/kg in the muscle, liver, lung, heart, kidney and brain, respectively, within the first 5 days after application. The eggs from hens treated externally with 6-8% trichlorfon contained trichlorfon levels of 0.01-0.05 mg/kg (IRPTC/GKNT, 1983).

Residues of trichlorfon one day after the spraying of chickens at the rate of 150 mg/kg body weight were as follows (mg/kg): egg shell, 0.48; egg white, 0.27; egg yolk, not detectable. Trichlorfon was preserved in chicken carcasses kept for six months at -10 °C, but it quickly decomposed when the carcasses were boiled (Dmitriyev, 1970).

5.2.5 *Fish*

Trichlorfon residues in eels were determined 1 and 5 days after ponds were treated with a 1 mg/litre aqueous solution of the insecticide. The results showed that the insecticide decomposed in a short time to form dichlorvos in neutral and weakly alkaline water. In pond water with a pH of 8-10, less than 10% of the applied trichlorfon was degraded after 30 min and dichlorvos was detected. The residues of trichlorfon and dichlorvos in the eels were 0.009-0.032 mg/kg and <0.005-0.02 mg/kg, respectively, on the first day following treatment, and 0.011 mg/kg and 0.009-0.032 mg/kg, respectively, on the 4th day after treatment. There was a good correlation between the residual amounts of trichlorfon in the eels and the concentrations in the water. Residues of trichlorfon and dichlorvos, which were detected on the skin of eels in water at pH 7.0, could be removed by rinsing. Insecticide residues were found in the internal organs of only one out of 7 eels caught in the field pond. Carps exposed to an aqueous solution of trichlorfon at 0.25 mg/kg were examined on the 2nd, 4th, and 9th days after exposure. Residues of trichlorfon and dichlorvos could not be detected in the fish on the second day (Nakahara et al., 1973).

5.3 Occupational exposure

A thousand-fold dilution of 50% trichlorfon emulsifiable concentrate was applied to apple trees by operators using a speed sprayer or a power sprayer; the operators wore their usual working clothes or special protective clothes, plus rubber gloves, full length rubber boots, and masks with, or without, charcoal filters. The plasma and red blood cell cholinesterase activity of the operators following both kinds of spraying did not show any significant changes compared with pre-exposure values. The calculated cumulative trichlorfon exposures per person with a speed sprayer and a power sprayer were 177 $\pm$ 54.0 mg and 1179 $\pm$ 398 mg, respectively (Kawai et al., 1982).

Occupational exposures to levels exceeding 0.5 mg/m^3 have been reported (Lu et al., 1984; Hu et al., 1986).

6. KINETICS AND METABOLISM

6.1 Absorption and distribution

6.1.1 Animal

In cattle, percutaneous absorption of ^{32}P-labelled trichlorfon after pour-on application is extremely affected by the solvent used (Dedek & Schwarz, 1967). With a 2% aqueous solution, only very little trichlorfon ended up in the blood (about 0.15 mg/litre). In contrast, trichlorfon in a 2% mineral oil solution, was absorbed rapidly, reaching a maximum concentration in the blood of 3.1 mg/litre at 42 min. The percutaneous absorption rate was considerably slower in sheep, than in cattle (Dedek & Schwarz, 1970). In *in vitro* absorption studies on isolated cattle skin, partition of trichlorfon was dependent on the relative solubilities in the water (blood) and organic phases (Dedek & Schwarz, 1967).

Trichlorfon administered orally to mammals is rapidly absorbed, degraded, and eliminated. When ^{32}P-labelled trichlorfon was administered orally to a cow (25 mg/kg), the radioactivity appeared in the blood within half an hour and reached a maximum (15.1 mg/litre trichlorfon equivalent) between 1 and 3 h. It, then decreased rapidly (less than 1 mg/litre) within 24 h of treatment (Robbins et al., 1956). In the liver and brain of a mouse treated orally with ^{32}P-trichlorfon (6.2 mg/mouse), chloroform extractable radioactivity of 188 mg/kg and 28.2 mg/kg trichlorfon equivalents, respectively, was found, 15 min after treatment (Miyata & Saito, 1973). The radioactivity decreased rapidly to 6.4 and 1.61 mg/kg trichlorfon equivalents, respectively, at 4 h. The biological half-life of trichlorfon in mice was about 80 min, when it was administered orally.

Thirty minutes after radiolabelled trichlorfon was given by stomach tube to pregnant guinea-pigs on days 35 and 52 of gestation, the compound had rapidly become distributed to the main organs of the animals, the highest concentrations being present in the liver, kidney, and lung. Thirty minutes after dosing, there was a substantial uptake of trichlorfon into the fetus, and this became more pronounced at the later stage of gestation (52 days), the concentration in fetal liver equalling that in the placenta at that time (Berge & Nafstad, 1986).

6.1.2 Human

In the blood of a patient who ingested 10 g of trichlorfon, the concentration of the insecticide was 270 μg/litre after 24 h, following which it rapidly decreased and was undetectable after 94 h (Fournier et al., 1978). In a 70-year-old woman who died from acute trichlorfon poisoning, caused by the ingestion of a 50% emulsifiable concentrate, the levels of trichlorfon in the organs (μg/g) were 310 in the blood, 487 in the liver, 465 in the brain, 416 in the kidney, and 2240 in the urine. In addition, about 7.2 g of trichlorfon was found in the stomach contents (Yashiki et al., 1982).

A 76-year-old male, who had attempted suicide by ingesting about 50 ml of trichlorfon, died approximately 8 h later. The trichlorfon concentration was found to be 215 μg/g in a blood sample and 15.0 mg/g in a gastric lavage liquid sample, both of which were collected about 1 h after intake (Yashiki et al., 1988).

Following the administration of metrifonate to humans at doses of 7.5-10 mg/kg body weight, peak levels of trichlorfon in the plasma (8 μg/ml) were reached in 2 h or less. Detectable levels were still present in the body after 8 h (Nordgren, 1981).

Four groups of 4 healthy human volunteers each were given metrifonate at 2.5, 5, 7.5, or 15 mg/kg (single dose). Peak plasma levels of 5-10, 5-15, 10-25, or 15-100 μmol/litre were observed after each of the respective doses. There was no evidence of dose-dependent kinetics (Aden Abdi, 1990).

6.2 Biotransformation

Trichlorfon(1) rearranges readily to form dichlorvos (2,2-dichlorovinyl dimethyl phosphate)(2) via dehydrochlorination (Lorenz et al., 1955; Metcalf et al., 1959; Nordgren et al., 1978; Hofer, 1981; Nordgren, 1981). This transformation occurs under physiological conditions (Miyamoto, 1959). Dichlorvos has been found in animal tissues *in vivo* at less than 5% of the administered dose following trichlorfon treatment (Metcalf et al., 1959; Nordgren et al., 1978; Dedek, 1981). However, it could not be detected very often and only its degradation products, such as demethyl dichlorvos (2,2-dichlorovinyl methyl hydrogen phosphate)(4) were found, as evidence of the formation of dichlorvos *in vivo* (Arthur & Casida,

1957; Bull & Ridgway, 1969; Miyata & Saito, 1973; Otto et al., 1980). Dichlorvos is also formed from trichlorfon in humans. Following the administration of metrifonate, dichlorvos was found in erythrocytes and plasma at levels corresponding to 0.2-1% of the metrifonate concentrations (Nordgren, 1981; Aden Abdi, 1990).

In *in vitro* experiments, the conversion of trichlorfon into dichlorvos was demonstrated by incubating with serum (Dedek & Schwarz, 1966), with the soluble fraction from cow and chicken liver homogenates (Akhtar, 1982), and with the digestive juice of the silkworm larvae (Sugiyama & Shigematsu, 1969). Demethylation also occurred with liver homogenates. The half-life of trichlorfon in the blood of various mammals *in vitro* ranged up to 30 min (Dedek & Schwarz, 1966). Using housefly homogenate, another metabolite was produced with the same mass spectrum as dichlorvos, but a different R_f value on TLC; it was proposed that this was dimethyl 2,2-dichloro-1-hydroxyvinylphosphonate (Lange, 1980).

The main metabolites of ^{32}P-trichlorfon found in mammals were demethyl trichlorfon (Fig. 2)(6), demethyl dichlorvos(4), dimethyl hydrogen phosphate(5), methyl hydrogen phosphate(7) and phosphoric acid(8) (Hassan et al., 1965; Bull & Ridgway, 1969; Miyata & Saito, 1973). The percentages of the water-extractable metabolites found in the whole body in mice, 0.5 and 4 h after oral administration of 6.2 mg ^{32}P-trichlorfon, were, respectively, demethyl trichlorfon (4.3, 4.0), demethyl dichlorvos (20.8, 9.9), dimethyl hydrogen phosphate (34.6, 47.8), methyl hydrogen phosphate (14.3, 17.8), phosphoric acid (22.4, 20.9), and unknown compounds (3.6, 0.0) (Miyata & Saito, 1973).

The glucuronide of trichloroethanol(9) was isolated from the urine of a dog in amounts equivalent to 67% of the administered dose of trichlorfon, indicating the occurrence of hydrolytic P-C bond cleavage (Arthur & Casida, 1957). Another glucuronide containing phosphorus and chlorine atoms in 1:2 ratio was found in the urine of rabbits administered with trichlorfon (Miyamoto, 1961).

Thus, the main degradation routes of trichlorfon are demethylation, P-C bond cleavage, and ester hydrolysis via dichlorvos. Proposed metabolic pathways of trichlorfon, together with the established metabolic pathways of dichlorvos, are illustrated in Fig. 2.

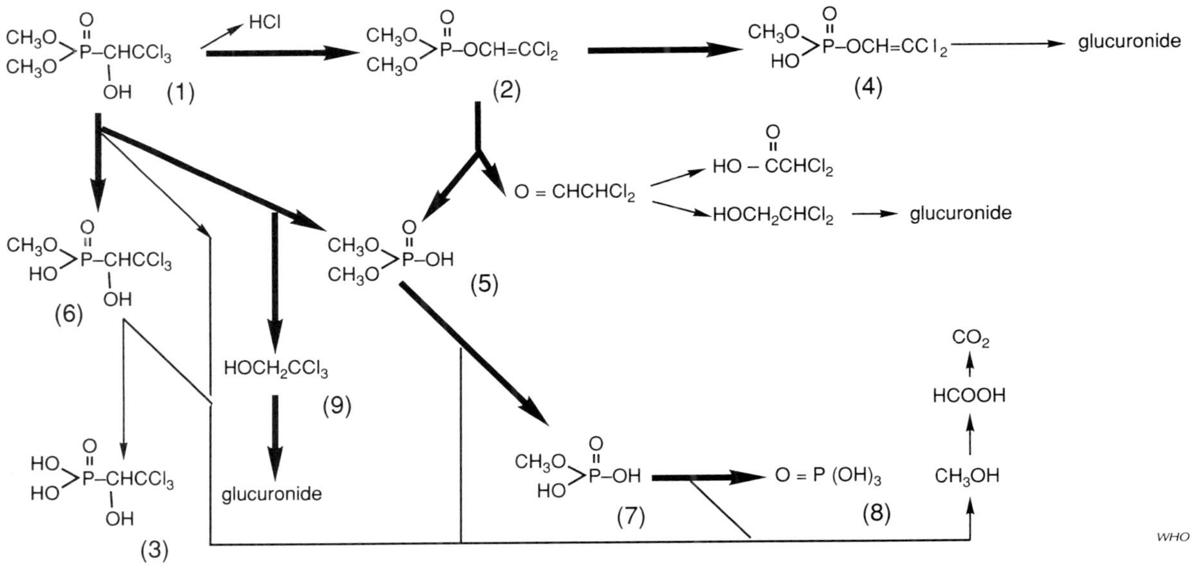

WHO 91710

Fig. 2. Proposed metabolic pathways for trichlorfon.

6.3 Elimination and excretion

Trichlorfon administered to mammals is rapidly eliminated, primarily via the urine. About 66% of the dose administered orally to cows was eliminated in the urine within 12 h. Following oral administration (6.2 mg/animal) of ^{32}P-trichlorfon to mice, 70% of the total dose was eliminated in the urine and faeces in 12 h (Miyata & Saito, 1973). More than 80% of the eliminated compound was present in the urine. The majority of the eliminated radioactive compounds in both the urine and faeces were degradation products, and only a small percentage of them were chloroform extractable. The biological half-life of trichlorfon administered orally to mice was estimated to be about 80 min (Robbins et al., 1956).

When methyl-^{14}C-trichlorfon was administered intraperitoneally to rats, 24% of the radioactive carbon was eliminated as carbon dioxide in the expired air, within 10 h; 32% was present in the urine as formate and dimethyl hydrogen phosphate, within 24 h (Hassan & Zayed, 1965).

Residues of trichlorfon were detected in the milk following the oral treatment of cows. Less than 0.2% of the total dose administered was recovered in the milk at the end of 144 h (Robbins et al., 1956). Single doses of 3 or 30 mg/kg body weight resulted in maximum residues in the milk of 0.09 mg/kg in 3 h and 0.55 mg/kg in 1 h, respectively; the residues then decreased rapidly to 0.003-0.007 mg/kg at 24 h. A small amount of dichlorvos (0.04 mg/kg) was detected as a metabolite in the milk, 1-3 h after the higher dose (Nakahara et al., 1972). When lactating cows were treated dermally by washing with 11.2% trichlorfon, 6-8 h before milking, trichlorfon residues (equal to or more than 0.2 mg/kg) and dichlorvos residues (0.03 mg/kg) were found in the first milking (Fechner et al., 1968). Trichlorfon was detected up to the third milking, 32 h after application, but neither trichlorfon nor dichlorvos could be demonstrated in the fourth milking.

6.4 Reaction with body components

6.4.1 In vitro *studies*

Several investigators have reported the considerable inhibitory activity of trichlorfon on acetylcholinesterase *in vitro*. The pI_{50} for acetylcholinesterase was 5.5 and the bimolecular rate constant for rat brain acetylcholinesterase was 3.18 × 10^4/min (Arthur & Casida, 1957; Buchet & Lauwerys, 1970). The activity is, however, strongly pH-dependent and is about 30-fold more active at pH 7.4-7.6 than at pH 6.0-6.5. At the lower pH range, trichlorfon is more stable with practically no inhibiting activity against cholinesterases. In contrast, dichlorvos is equally active at this pH range (Metcalf et al., 1959; Miyamoto 1959; Reiner et al., 1975). However, the rates of non-enzymatic reactivation of the enzymes after inhibition by trichlorfon and dichlorvos are similar. Thus, it is now believed that the *in vitro* inhibitory activity of trichlorfon is due to its rapid, spontaneous, non-enzymatic conversion into dichlorvos.

Frohlich et al. (1990) determined the competitive and uncompetitive constants for the action of trichlorfon on bee *p*-nitrophenyl acetate hydrolysing esterase to be 4.5 × 10^{-6} mol/litre and 1.6 × 10^{-5} mol/litre, respectively.

The inhibition constant for trichlorfon and chicken liver fluoracetanilidase was determined to be 2.5 × 10^{-6} mol/litre (Nakamura & Ueda, 1967).

6.4.2 In vivo *studies*

In rats given trichlorfon intraperitoneally at 150 mg/kg, considerable increases in the activities of superoxide dismutase (× 1.94) and microsomal cytochrome P-450 (× 2.09), and in lipid peroxidation (× 1.44) in the liver were observed, 2.5 h after treatment (Matkovics et al., 1980).

In *in vivo* studies on mice receiving a diet containing 100 mg trichlorfon/kg, the cholinesterase activities in the brain, erythrocytes, and plasma were, respectively, 72.1, 115.7, and 92.7% of control values after one-day (24 h) and 79.9, 83.8, and 81.0%, respectively, after 20 days (Tsumuki et al., 1970).

A mixture of trichlorfon and phenothiazine, which was administered to horses with feed as an antihelminthic at a single dose level of 35.8 mg/kg, reduced the cholinesterase activity in whole blood and plasma to 32 and 20%, respectively, by 24 h. The activity increased to about 80% after 4 weeks (Bello et al., 1974).

In humans who received an oral dose of 7.5 mg trichlorfon/kg on two successive days, the maximum inhibition of erythrocyte and plasma cholinesterase was 52 and 94%, respectively. The red cell cholinesterase activity recovered very slowly to reach only 66% of the pretreatment level, 28 days after treatment, while that of the plasma cholinesterase recovered rapidly to reach 78% at 22 days (Lebrun & Cerf, 1960).

When $^{14}CH_3$-labelled trichlorfon was adminstered intravenously to rats at 40 mg/kg, the radioactive carbon (^{14}C) was found mainly in the liver (25 mg/kg) and kidneys (11.6 mg/kg), 3 h after treatment (Dedek & Lohs, 1970). Similar results were obtained with intra-peritoneal treatment. Only about 1% of the radioactivity found in the organs was extractable with acetone, indicating that most of the ^{14}C in the tissues was bound to body components. The bound ^{14}C in the organs investigated was less than 10% of the total dose. It disappeared rather rapidly and the bound radioactivity decreased to about one-tenth by 17 h. In another study, about 10% of the phosphorus portion, administered orally to mice as ^{32}P-trichlorfon, was found bound to tissue (Miyata & Saito, 1973).

7. EFFECTS ON ORGANISMS IN THE ENVIRONMENT

Acute toxicity data for trichlorfon on aquatic and terrestrial non-target organisms are summarized in Tables 8 and 9, respectively.

7.1 Microorganisms

When trichlorfon was applied to a cotton field at 0.5 g/m^2, the total count of soil fungi and the counts of some fungal species, such as *Aspergillus niger*, *Fusarium oxysporum*, and *A. fumigatus* were elevated 3 days after treatment. A depressed effect was observed in *Myrothecium verrucaria*. After 40 days, trichlorfon did not have any significant effects on the total count of soil fungi (Abdel-Kader et al., 1978). Trichlorfon at 8-16 mg/kg in agar affected the mycelial growth of 4 fungi (*A. fumigatus*, *F. moniliforme*, *Penicillium italicum*, and *Sclerotium cepivorum*), even 10 days after application (El-Hissy & Abdel-Kader, 1980).

In field pond trials, Grygierek & Wasilewska (1981) found that trichlorfon applied at 1 mg/litre reduced zooplankton numbers within the first 24 h of application and bottom fauna after 1 week. Rotifers (*Keratella* sp.) and cladocerans (*Bosmina*) were especially sensitive to the chemical. The renewal of the affected fauna communities took about 1 month. When the pond was treated with trichlorfon at 300-800 μg/litre, the numbers of cladocerans and copepods decreased, whereas rotifers and phytoplankton increased markedly in number. However, the total biomass was not affected (Grahl et al., 1981).

Cain & Cain (1984) incubated the green alga *Chlamydomonas moewusii* in a medium containing trichlorfon at concentrations up to 80 μmol/litre (21 mg/litre). At the highest concentration, growth of the algae was 76% of control levels. Zygospore germination of *Chlamydomonas* was unaffected at 80 μmol/litre (21 mg/litre) (108% of controls).

7.2 Invertebrates

Trichlorfon is highly toxic for aquatic arthropods with LC_{50} values ranging from 0.75 to 7800 μg/litre in 48-/96-h tests (Table 8).

Table 8. Acute toxicity of trichlorfon for non-target aquatic organisms

Species	Size	Toxicity	(mg/litre)	Formulation[a]	System[b]	Temperature (°C)	pH	Hardness[c]	Reference
Protozoa									
Colpidium campylum		MAD	10			20			Dive et al. (1980)
Fish									
Rainbow trout (*Salmo gairdneri*)		96-h LC_{50}	4.85	T	S	12			Marking & Mauck (1975)
Cutthroat trout (*Salmo clarki*)		96-h LC_{50}	1.68	T	S	12	7.5	40	Woodward & Mauck (1980)
		96-h LC_{50}	3.25	T	S	12	7.5	40	
		96-h LC_{50}	5.75	T	S	7	7.5	40	
		96-h LC_{50}	4.75	T	S	12	6.5	40	
		96-h LC_{50}	0.375	T	S	12	8.5	40	
		96-h LC_{50}	0.620	T	S	12	7.8	320	
Cherry salmon (*Onchorhyncus masou*)	2.8 g	12-h LC_{50}	10.2	50%EC	SS	17.6			Kimura et al. (1971)
	2.8 g	24-h LC_{50}	1.1	50%EC	SS	17.6			
	2.8 g	48-h LC_{50}	1.1	50%EC	SS	17.6			
	2.8 g	96-h LC_{50}	1.1	50%EC	SS	17.6			
Carp (*Cyprinus carpio*)	egg	24-h LC_{50}	15	EC	S	25	6.9-7.2		Hashimoto et al. (1982)
	0.60 cm	24-h LC_{50}	11	EC	S	25	6.9-7.2		
	0.73 cm	24-h LC_{50}	8.8	EC	S	25	6.9-7.2		
	1.16 cm, 0.013 g	24-h LC_{50}	14	EC	S	25	6.9-7.2		
	1.52 cm, 0.038 g	24-h LC_{50}	15	EC	S	25	6.9-7.2		
	2.51 cm, 0.23 g	24-h LC_{50}	14	EC	S	25	6.9-7.2		
	3.86 cm, 0.87 g	24-h LC_{50}	15	EC	S	25	6.9-7.2		
	5.22 cm, 2.34 g	24-h LC_{50}	15	EC	S	25	6.9-7.2		

Table 8. (continued)

Carp (*Cyprinus carpio*)		48-h LC_{50}	1200	4%D	S	25			Nishiuchi (1979a)
		48-h LC_{50}	30	50%EC	S	25			
		48-h LC_{50}	50	80%WP	S	25			
Carp (*Cyprinus carpio*)	5.3 cm, 2.2 g	24-h LC_{50}	40		S	15			Nishiuchi (1977)
	5.3 cm, 2.2 g	24-h LC_{50}	40		S	20			
	5.3 cm, 2.2 g	24-h LC_{50}	28		S	25			
	5.3 cm, 2.2 g	24-h LC_{50}	25		S	30			
	5.3 cm, 2.2 g	24-h LC_{50}	25		S	35			
Fathead minnow (*Pimephales promelas*)		96-h LC_{50}	51						Livingston (1977)
American eel (*Anguilla rostrata*)	black stage	96-h LC_{50}	1.32		S	22	7.2-7.6	40-48	Spehar et al. (1981)
	glass stage	96-h LC_{50}	1.31		S	22	7.2-7.6	40-48	
	yellow phase	96-h LC_{50}	8.57		S	22	7.2-7.6	40-48	Hinton & Eversole (1980)
Striped bass (*Roccus saxatilis*)	6 cm, 2.7 g	24-h LC_{50}	10.4	50%SP	S	21	8.2	35	Wellborn Jr. (1969)
	6 cm, 2.7 g	48-h LC_{50}	9.2	50%SP	S	21	8.2	35	
	6 cm, 2.7 g	96-h LC_{50}	5.2	50%SP	S	21	8.2	35	
Bluegill (*Lepomis macrochirus*)	0.87-2.4 g	24-h LC_{50}	41.0[a]	50%SP	S	18	7	51.3	McCann & Jasper (1972)

Table 8. (continued)

Species	Size	Toxicity	(mg/litre)	Formulation[a]	System[b]	Temperature (°C)	pH	Hardness[c]	Reference
Arthropods									
Water flea (*Daphnia pulex*)		3-h LC_{50}	0.18	4%P	S	25			Nishiuchi (1979b)
		3-h LC_{50}	0.030	50%EC	S	25			
		3-h LC_{50}	0.019	80%WP	S	25			
Water flea (*Daphnia carinata*)		1-h LC_{50}	0.088	EC	S	25			Nishiuchi (1979c)
		3-h LC_{50}	0.014	EC	S	25			
		6-h LC_{50}	0.0064	EC	S	25			
		24-h LC_{50}	0.0012	EC	S	25			
		48-h LC_{50}	0.00075	EC	S	25			
Amphipod (*Gammarus pseudolimnaeus*)		96-h LC_{50}	0.108	T	S	12	7.5	40	Woodward & Mauck (1980)
		96-h LC_{50}	0.052	T	S	12	8.5	40	
Mayfly (*Cloeon diptrum*)	9.3 mm, 5.6 mg	3-h LC_{50}	1.8	EC	S	25			Nishiuchi & Asano (1979)
	9.3 mm, 5.6 mg	6-h LC_{50}	0.75	EC	S	25			
	9.3 mm, 5.6 mg	24-h LC_{50}	0.075	EC	S	25			
	9.3 mm, 5.6 mg	48-h LC_{50}	0.056	EC	S	25			
Dragon fly (*Orthetrum albistylum speciosum*)	2.3 cm, 0.62 g	48-h LC_{50}	0.042	EC		25			Nishiuchi (1981)
(*Sympetrum frequens*)	2.1 cm, 0.56 g	48-h LC_{50}	0.15	EC		25			Nishiuchi (1981)
(*Sigara substriata*)	5.9 mm, 6.1 mg	48-h LC_{50}	0.15	EC		25			Nishiuchi (1981)

Table 8. (continued)

(*Micronecta sedula*)	3.2 mm, 1.8 mg	48-h LC_{50}	0.075	EC		25			Nishiuchi (1981)
Stonefly		96-h LC_{50}	0.100	T	S	12	8.5	40	Woodward &
(*Pteronarcella badia*)		96-h LC_{50}	0.0098	T	S	12	7.5	40	Mauck
		96-h LC_{50}	0.0053	T	S	12	6.5	40	(1980)
(*Eretes sticticus*)	1.5 cm, 0.20 g	48-h LC_{50}	0.32	EC		25			Nishiuchi (1981)
Crayfish (*Procambarus clarkii*)	adults, 15-38 g	96-h LC_{50}	7.8	T	S	19	7.8	35	Andreu-Moliner (1986)
Mollusca									
Snail (*Semisulcospira libertina*)	2.9 cm, 1.6 g	48-h LC_{50}	1.8	EC		22			Nishiuchi & Yoshida (1972)
Snail (*Cipangopaludina malleata*)	2.4 cm, 3.3 g	48-h LC_{50}	4.8	EC		22			Nishiuchi & Yoshida (1972)
Red snail (*Indoplanorbis exustus*)	0.72 cm. 1.1 g	48-h LC_{50}	1.8	EC		22			Nishiuchi & Yoshida (1972)
Physa-snail (*Physa acuta*)	0.91 cm, 0.11 g	48-h LC_{50}	3.2	EC		22			Nishiuchi & Yoshida (1972)
		10-day LC_{50}	0.05			15-20	7.3		Mandoul et al. (1967)

Table 8. (continued)

Species	Size	Toxicity	(mg/litre)	Formulation[a]	System[b]	Temperature (°C)	pH	Hardness[c]	Reference
Snail (*Lymnaea acuminata*)	1.2 cm	48-h LC_{50}	2.2						Singh & Agarwal (1981)
	1.2 cm	72-h LC_{50}	0.65						
	1.2 cm	96-h LC_{50}	0.3						
	1.2 cm	168-h LC_{50}	0.22						
	1.2 cm	240-h LC_{50}	0.058						
(*Pila globosa*)	3.5 cm	48-h LC_{50}	25.4						Singh & Agarwal (1981)
	3.5 cm	72-h LC_{50}	19.0						
	3.5 cm	96-h LC_{50}	8.0						
	3.5 cm	168-h LC_{50}	2.8						
	3.5 cm	240-h LC_{50}	2.2						
(*Gryphaea angulata*)		10-day LC_{50}	2.45			9-19		SW	Mandoul et al. (1967)

[a] T = Technical.
EC = Emulsifiable concentrate.
D = Dust.
WP = Wettable powder.
SP = Soluble powder.
P = Powder.

[b] S = Static.
SS = Semi-static.
SW = Sea water.
MAD = Minimal active dose.

[c] Hardness (mg/litre as $CaCO_3$).

The toxicity of trichlorfon for amphipods increased 2-fold when the pH of the media was increased from 7.5 to 8.5; similarly the toxicity for stonefly naiads increased about 20-fold when the pH was increased from 6.5 to 8.5 (Woodward & Mauck, 1980). Trichlorfon is less toxic for mollusca, the 48-h LC_{50} values ranging up to 25.4 mg/litre. Prolonged exposure (10 days) resulted in a 10-40 times increase in toxicity (Singh & Agarwal, 1981).

Trichlorfon at concentrations of up to 30 mg/litre did not affect byssal attachment in seed mussels (*Mytilus edulis*) (Roberts, 1975).

Trichlorfon showed cholinomimetic properties on the excitor or inhibitor receptors of acetylcholine in the isolated heart, median dorsal radula protractor muscle, and rectum of the snail *Pila globosa* (Singh & Agarwal, 1979).

When freshwater snail, *Lymnaea acuminata*, was exposed to 10 or 20 mg trichlorfon/litre for 48 h, the rate of oxygen consumption and the concentration of glycogen were both reduced, while the levels of lactic acid and reducing sugars were enhanced. The effects persisted for 7 days after withdrawal of the trichlorfon. On the basis of these observations, Mahendru & Agarwal (1981) concluded that trichlorfon may affect not only cholinesterase activity but also other enzyme systems, such as the ones involved in carbohydrate metabolism.

7.3 Aquatic vertebrates

Trichlorfon is moderately toxic for fish, the 96-h LC_{50} values ranging from 0.4 to 51 mg/litre (Table 8). The effects of trichlorfon on the susceptibility of the developmental stages of carp were not remarkable (Hashimoto et al., 1982). However, with regard to water quality, the toxicity for fish increased as the water temperature, pH, and hardness increased. The increase in toxicity was affected least (3.4 fold) by increasing the temperature from 7 to 12 °C and most (13-fold) by changing the pH from 6.5 to 8.5 (Woodward & Mauck, 1980).

Cherry salmon fingerlings (*Onchorhyncus masou*) were exposed to one-tenth (0.105 mg/litre) and one-third (0.310 mg/litre) of the 96-h LC_{50} value (1.1 mg/litre) of trichlorfon for 6 weeks in a flow-through system. Trichlorfon initially retarded the growth of the fish at both concentrations, but then the fish grew normally, and the condition factors (weight-length coefficent) of the test fish did not differ significantly from those of the controls after 6 weeks of exposure to trichlorfon. Histopathological examination showed that the liver cells were swollen with an obscure cell contour at the beginning of the study, but no compound-induced histopathological changes were observed after 6 weeks of exposure (Kimura et al., 1971).

When bluegill fingerlings were exposed to formulations of trichlorfon, haemorrhage along, and fractures of, the caudal vertebrae (usually extended over three vertebrae) occurred 4-8 h after treatment at concentrations of 8-52 mg/litre (McCann & Jasper, 1972).

Matton & Laham (1969) treated 1-inch rainbow trout larvae for 16 h with 10-100 mg trichlorfon/litre, or for 40 h with 5 mg/litre. Histochemical examination revealed that the acetylcholinesterase activity was inhibited in the septa of the myotomes and at the myoneural junctions. Furthermore, pathological changes were observed in the heart, liver, blood cells, pseudogills, and muscular tissues.

7.4 Terrestrial vertebrates

Trichlorfon is relatively toxic for birds with oral LD_{50} values of 40-180 mg/kg body weight (Table 9). Peakall & Bart (1983) reported a 5-day LD_{50} value of 720 mg/kg for Bobwhite quail.

Residues of trichlorfon and dichlorvos in the bodies of canopy-feeder birds (Baltimore orioles, crested fly-catcher, and blue jay) were 0.005-0.04 mg/kg, 3 days following an aerial application of trichlorfon at 1.12 kg/ha (Kurtz & Studholme, 1974).

Following aerial spraying of trichlorfon at 1.12 kg/ha, the brain cholinesterase activity was about 20% less than that in the controls in 2 out of 10 bird-species; in the other 8 species, the activity was not depressed, even immediately after spraying (Zinkl et al., 1977).

According to a survey based on two, 1-h counts in 20-ha plots, 5 days before and after the spraying of 1120 g trichlorfon/ha, a virtually identical change in the number of bird species and the total number of hearings was observed. The application of trichlorfon resulted in a slight drop in song-bird activity (165 to 151). It did not produce any effects on cholinesterase activity in fly-catchers and only

Table 9. Acute toxicity of trichlorfon for non-target terrestrial organisms

Species	Size	Application	Toxicity		Formulation[a]	Temperature (°C)	Reference
Birds							
Red-winged blackbird (*Agelaius phoeniceus*)		oral	LD_{50}	37-75 mg/kg			Schafer Jr et al. (1983)
		oral	LD_{50}	40 mg/kg			Schafer (1972)
European starling (*Sturnus vulgaris*)		oral	LD_{50}	43 mg/kg			Schafer Jr et al. (1983)
		oral	LD_{50}	47 mg/kg			Schafer (1972)
(*Columbia livia*)	250-380 g	oral	LD_{50}	179.9 mg/kg			Hattori (1974)
White leghorn hen	1.5-2.0 kg	oral intraperitoneal	LD_{50} LD_{50}	75 mg/kg 75 mg/kg			Kimmerle & Löser (1974)
Japanese quail (*Coturnix coturnix japonica*)		oral	LD_{50}	50 mg/kg			Gromysz-Kalkowska (1985)

Table 9. (continued)

Species	Size	Application	Toxicity		Formulation[a]	Temperature (°C)	Reference
Arthropods							
Honey-bee (*Apis mellifera*, L)		sprayed on glass plate	LC_{50}	0.600 W/V%			Abdelwahab et al. (1973)
		weathered residues (3 h)	24-h	17% mortality	50%SP	26	Johansen (1972)
	128.6 mg	topical	LD_{50}	28.5 μg/g	T	16	Ahmad & Johansen (1973)
Alfalfa leafcutter bee (*Megachile rotundate*, F)		weathered residues (3 h)	24-h	5% mortality	50%SP	31	Johansen (1972)
	22.2 mg	topical	LD_{50}	250 μg/g	T	16	Ahmad &
	26.1 mg		LD_{50}	515 μg/g	T	16	Johansen (1973)
Alkali bee (*Nomia melanderi*, Cockerell)		weathered residues (3 h)	24-h	31% mortality	50%SP	31	Johansen (1972)

[a] SP = Soluble powder.
T = Technical grade.

10% inhibition in northern oriols, after 3 days. There was a considerable decrease in the singing of male birds after spraying; a marked increase in feeding activity immediately following spraying was noted. However, examination of the data on individual species does not show any consistent pattern: the great crested fly-catcher decreased but other fly-catchers did not, the American redstart decreased, but another canopy species, the red-eyed vireo, did not. No significant effects on the numbers of breeding pairs, bird abundance, nesting success, or mortality were found. Brain ChE levels were reduced by 20% in 6 out of 103 birds collected during the 5-day period following spray (Peakall & Bart, 1983).

Japanese quail were given trichlorfon daily for 20 days at an oral dose of 5 mg/kg body weight. Haematological examinations were made on the 5th, 10th, 15th, and 20th day of treatment and on the 5th, 10th, 15th, and 30th day after stopping treatment. The number of erythrocytes dropped on the 5th and 10th days, and the values of the haematocrit and haemoglobin fell on the 5th day. A significant increase in erythroblast contents was found on the 5th and 10th day. No other significant changes of the above parameters were observed up to the 30th day after treatment. The numbers of leukocytes, lymphocytes, neutrophils, and monocytes sharply increased from the 5th to 15th day of treatment, and quickly dropped to normal ranges on the 10th day after stopping treatment (Gromysz-Kalkowska et al., 1985).

7.5 Ecosystems

Trichlorfon applied to ponds at the rate of 1 mg/litre water destroyed the food invertebrates for fish. Large numbers of zooplankton, rotifers, and crustacea, died in the first 24 h after treatment, whereas benthos died during the first week. The affected fauna, community recovered slowly. Trichlorfon treatment deprived the fish of valuable foods, such as crustacean and bottom fauna, for as long as 1 month after treatment (Grygierek & Wasilewska, 1981).

8. EFFECTS ON EXPERIMENTAL ANIMALS AND *IN VITRO* TEST SYSTEMS

A more complete treatise on the effects of organophosphorus insecticides in general, especially their short- and long-term effects on the nervous system, will be found in the WHO Environmental Health Criteria 63: Organophosphorus insecticides - A general introduction (WHO, 1986).

No-observed-effect levels in animals treated with trichlorfon under various conditions are summarized in Annex II.

8.1 Acute toxicity

LD_{50} values for trichlorfon in different species and following different routes of administration are shown in Table 10. Species differences in LD_{50} values seem to be rather small.

Table 10. Acute toxicity of trichlorfon for several animal species

Animal	Sex	Route	Parameter	Value	Reference
Mouse	M	oral	LD_{50}	800 mg/kg	Haley et al. (1975)
	F			800 mg/kg	
	M	ip	LD_{50}	600 mg/kg	Soliman et al. (1984)
Rat	M	oral	LD_{50}	660 mg/kg	Benes & Cerna (1970)
	M	oral	LD_{50}	630 mg/kg	Gaines (1969)
	F			560 mg/kg	
	M,F	dermal	LD_{50}	> 2000 mg/kg	
	M	dermal	LD_{50}	2800 mg/kg	Edson & Noakes (1960)
	M	ip (23-day old)	LD_{50}	190 mg/kg	Brodeur & Dubois (1963)
		ip (adult)		250 mg/kg	
	M,F	inhalation (4 h)	LC_{50}	533 mg/m^3	Kimmerle (1975a)
Guinea-pig	M,F	ip	LD_{50}	300 mg/kg	DuBois & Cotter (1955)
Rabbit	M	dermal	LD_{50}	5000 mg/kg	Deichmann & Lampe (1955)
Dog	M	oral	LD_{50}	420 mg/kg	Deichmann & Lampe (1955)

The acute toxicity of trichlorfon is due to the inhibition of acetylcholinesterase at the nerve endings by the degradation product dichlorvos, leading to accumulation of endogenous acetylcholine. The effects are manifested by muscarinic and central nervous system signs and symptoms (Taylor, 1980). In the rat, the toxic effects produced by trichlorfon are characteristics of organophosphorus poisoning, i.e., muscular fibrillation, salivation, lacrimation, incontinence, diarrhoea, respiratory distress, prostration, gasping, tonic and clonic convulsion, coma, and death. Trichlorfon caused rapid onset of poisoning, effects occurring within 5 min at approximate LD_{50} doses (Edson & Noakes, 1960).

Only a slight increase in mortality was noted in weanling Holtzman rats compared with that in adults, when treated with trichlorfon (Brodeur & DuBois, 1963).

Trichlorfon has a low dermal toxicity (LD_{50}: > 2000 mg/kg) compared with that of dichlorvos (LD_{50}: 75-900 mg/kg). The difference in lipid solubility between the two compounds may be a major factor accounting for this difference (Holmstedt et al., 1978).

Since trichlorfon is used as a parasiticide in livestock, studies have been conducted to assess the effects of the chemical on cholinesterase activity and clinical conditions. Administration to horses of a single dose of trichlorfon of 60 or 80 mg/kg body weight, by stomach tube, resulted in moderately severe and severe colic, respectively, whereas a single dose of 80 mg/kg mixed into the feed was associated with only a transient softening of the faeces. Doses of 40 mg/kg or less, by either method of administration, were generally tolerated without notable adverse effects except for the softening of the faeces, which tended to be self-limiting. Clinical trials at dose rates of 35-40 mg/kg in horses, including pregnant and nonpregnant mares, stallions, suckling and weanling foals, and yearlings, did not cause any notable adverse effects (Drudge et al., 1976).

Pretreatment of female and castrated male sheep with 1.5 mg trichlorfon/kg body weight by intravenous injection, which was insufficient to produce a significant depression of erythrocyte cholinesterase activity, produced toxic effects that were additive to those of coumaphos, subsequently administered at 4 mg/kg per day (Silvestri et al., 1975a,b).

Horses treated with trichlorfon (39.7 mg/kg body weight) combined with mebendazole (8.8 mg/kg body weight) did not show any, or only a few, side-effects, except ChE inhibition, whereas horses given higher dosages (up to 5 times this dose) showed dosage-related increases in the severity of clinical signs and inhibition of erythrocyte cholinesterase activity. Depression of the activity was detected within 1 h of treatment. The maximum depression ranged from 42% (at the initial dosage) to 75% (at a 5 times higher dosage). Recovery of base-line activity did not occur in any of the horses within 32 days after treatment (Gingerich & Mia, 1981).

8.2 Short-term exposure

Wistar albino rats (10 males per group) were fed trichlorfon at 0, 1, 5, 25, or 125 mg/kg diet for 16 weeks. Trichlorfon failed to cause erythrocyte cholinesterase depression at 125 mg/kg. No effects were noted on food consumption or growth, or during gross examination of the tissues (Edson & Noakes, 1960).

Rats (13/sex per group) were fed trichlorfon at dietary levels of 0, 20, 100, or 300 mg/kg diet for 16 weeks. Significant cholinesterase depression was noted at 300 mg/kg. No effects were observed at the 100 mg/kg level on growth, behaviour, food consumption, or on gross and microscopic examination of tissues (Doull & Dubois, 1956).

After oral administration of trichlorfon to guinea-pig (100 mg/kg body weight per day for 60 days) the haemoglobin content was decreased by 13.5% while the haematocrit value remained unchanged. Trichlorfon also decreased the serum cholinesterase activity by 50% and increased the activity of alkaline phosphatase by 36% (Krustev et al., 1976).

Two dogs were administered 45 mg trichlorfon/kg body weight, orally, for 6 days per week over 3 months. No cumulative effects were noted. The serum cholinesterase level was 60% of normal at the end of the study period. No deaths occurred (Deichmann & Lampe, 1955). In another study, dogs (one male and one female per group, 2 males and 2 females serving as controls) were fed trichlorfon at levels of 0, 50, 200, or 500 mg/kg diet for 12 weeks. Plasma and erythrocyte cholinesterase activity was depressed at 500 mg/kg diet and unaffected at 200 mg/kg diet. Recovery of enzyme activity was complete 6 weeks after the feeding of trichlorfon stopped (Williams et al., 1959).

Rats (10/sex per group) were exposed for 6 h a day over a 3-week period (total of 15 exposures) to an atmosphere containing trichlorfon at concentrations of 0, 12.7, 35.4, and 103.5 mg/m^3. Exposure to a concentration of 103.5 mg/m^3 slightly affected the health of the animals (no details available). Body weight gain, parameters of haematological and clinical chemistry examinations, and urinalyses were not influenced at any exposure level. Cholinesterase inhibition of 42, 31, and 22% was found in the plasma, erythrocytes, and the brain, respectively, in male animals at 103.5 mg/m^3; female animals showed dose-dependent inhibition values of 39, 26, and 26% at 35.4 mg/m^3 and 48, 44, and 47% at 103.5 mg/m^3 in the plasma, erythrocyte, and brain, respectively. The only significant alteration in relative organ weight was found in male animals showing dose-related increases in relative spleen weights of about 20 and 25% at the 35.4 and 103.5 mg/m^3 exposure levels, respectively. No abnormal histological findings were observed in any of the tissues examined microscopically (Kimmerle, 1975b).

In a 13-week study to evaluate target organ toxicity, dose-response, and maximum tolerated dose for a 2-year study, groups of 10 male and 10 female Fischer rats and B6C3F1 mice (8-week-old) were administered trichlorfon in the feed at 0, 62, 185, 555, 1666, or 5000 mg/kg, for 7 days a week. All the rats and mice survived the 13-week treatment, except one male mouse at 5000 mg/kg and one female mouse at 1666 mg/kg. The body weights of the 5000 mg/kg groups of male and female rats and mice were significantly lower compared with those of their respective controls. Plasma and erythrocyte cholinesterase activity was reduced in a dose-related manner in the rats and mice. Neurotoxicity tests showed that motor activity and grip strength were reduced in the 1666 and 5000 mg/kg groups of male and female rats and mice. No histo-pathological changes were observed in the brain, spinal cord, and sciatic nerve and other organ systems. Absolute and relative liver, kidney, and spleen weights were increased in the 1666 and 5000 mg/kg groups of male and female rats and mice. The weight increase was not accompanied by any histopathological findings. Two-year carcinogenicity studies on trichlorfon administered in the diet to male and female Fischer rats and B6C3F1 mice are in progress (Chan & Peters, 1989).

Groups of 7 male and 7 female Wistar rats were fed 1, 5, 10, 30, 50, or 100 mg trichlorfon/kg body weight in their diet for 12 weeks. A dose of 100 mg/kg, daily, inhibited the cholinesterase activity in all tissues examined, namely erythrocytes, serum, brain, heart, liver, and gastrocnemius muscle, but the extent of the inhibition differed between tissues. No significant histological changes were found in the parenchymatous organs, such as the brain, heart, lung, pituitary gland, thyroid gland, liver, intestine, stomach, kidney, adrenal gland, and testes. Despite the marked inhibition of the tissue cholinesterase activity in the treated animals, no changes were observed in nocturnal behaviour, reactivity to external stimuli, conjunctival and pinna reflexes, and the avoidance reflexes to painful stimuli (Shimamoto & Hattori, 1965).

Groups of 5 male and 5 female Rhesus monkeys (*Macaca mulatta*) were each administered technical trichlorfon by oral intubation at dose levels of 0, 0.1, or 0.2 mg/kg body weight per day for 26 weeks, in order to determine a no-observed-effect level on the cholinesterase activity in erythrocytes. There were no effects on appearance, behaviour, nutritional state, feed and water consumption, and body weight gain. No treatment-related changes were found in haematology, liver and kidney function, and erythrocyte cholinesterase activity. The NOEL in this study was 0.2 mg/kg body weight per day (Hoffmann et al., 1988).

8.3 Skin and eye irritation; sensitization

8.3.1 Skin irritation

A skin irritation test was conducted with technical trichlorfon applied to the intact and abraded skin of 6 albino rabbits. The contact time was 24 h and the animals were observed for 7 days. Technical trichlorfon did not irritate the skin (Thyssen, 1981).

Technical trichlorfon was tested on 6 New Zealand White rabbits for its dermal primary irritation potential. The test material was kept in contact with the shaved skin under an occlusion patch for 4 h, and scoring was performed for 72 h. The results indicated that technical trichlorfon is not a primary dermal irritant (Bond, 1986).

8.3.2 Skin sensitization

Technical trichlorfon was evaluated in a Magnusson and Kligman maximization test on guinea-pigs. The concentrations used were: intra-dermal induction, 1%; topical induction, 25%; first challenge, 25%; and second challenge, 12.5%. The results showed that technical trichlorfon is a sensitizer for guinea-pigs (Mihail, 1985).

Technical trichlorfon was investigated in the open epicutaneous test on guinea-pigs for skin-sensitizing potential. Induction (4 weeks, 5 days per week) was carried out using 0, 1, 3, or 10% test compound. Challenges were done with the same concentrations 4, 6, and 8 weeks after the start of the induction. The 3 and 10% dilutions of trichlorfon had a skin-sensitizing effect, but not the 1% dilution (Mihail, 1986a).

8.3.3 Eye irritation

An irritation test was performed using technical trichlorfon on 6 albino rats. The exposure times were 5 minutes and 24 h. Technical trichlorfon had a moderately irritating effect on the mucosae of the eye (Thyssen, 1981).

8.4 Long-term exposure

Several reviews on long-term toxicity studies on trichlorfon have been published (FAO/WHO, 1972, 1976, 1979; Holmstedt et al., 1978; Machemer, 1981; IARC, 1983).

8.4.1 Oral administration

8.4.1.1 Mouse

A group of 30 male and 28 female AB/Jena strain mice, 8 weeks of age, received 30 mg trichlorfon/kg body weight, by gavage, twice weekly for 75 weeks. A group of 30 male and 29 female mice served as controls. All surviving animals were killed in week 80. Inhibition of body weight gain and shortening of survival time were noted in the treated group. There was no statistically significant difference in the incidence of tumours between treated and control mice (Teichmann & Hauschild, 1978).

Groups of 60 male and 60 female Charles River CD-1 mice (6-week-old) were given 100, 300, or 1000 mg trichlorfon/kg diet for 90 weeks, except for males in the 1000 mg/kg group which were treated for 82 weeks. A group of 60 male and 60 female mice served as controls. Inhibition of body weight gain was observed in females given 300 or 1000 mg trichlorfon/kg diet. Cholinesterase activity was depressed in both sexes at 1000 mg/kg diet. The no-observed-effect level was 100 mg/kg diet. No significant microscopic alterations were reported. There was no statistically significant difference in the incidence of tumours between treated and control mice (Machemer, 1981).

Groups of 50 CD-1 mice per sex and dose level were given technical grade trichlorfon at 0, 300, 900, or 2700 mg/kg diet (analytical concentrations 0, 275, 891, or 2707 mg/kg diet) for 104 weeks. There were no significant differences between groups in feed consumption, haematological parameters, or mortality. Increased incidences of urine stain and ear lesions in males, and vaginal discharge in females, were regarded as non-specific cholinergic effects. The body weights of the 2700 mg/kg female mice were significantly increased throughout the study. There was a compound-related increase in liver weight in the 900 and 2700 mg/kg females with no corresponding light-microscopic changes, regarded as a compound-adaptive mechanism. All trichlorfon-treated groups showed significant blood cholinesterase depression throughout the study: 20%, in the 300 mg/kg females, and up to 74% in the 2700 mg/kg group; this latter dose was compatible with a maximum tolerated dose. No compound-related tumorigenicity was found in this study (Hayes, 1988).

8.4.1.2 *Rat*

Groups of 25 male and 25 female, 4-week-old, Sprague-Dawley rats were fed trichlorfon in the diet at doses of 0, 50, 250, 500, or 1000 mg/kg diet. The treatment continued for 17 months for the males and 24 months for the females. Survival time was shortened in both males and females given 1000 mg/kg diet. Retarded growth rate was observed in males given 1000 mg/kg diet: their weight was 15% less than the controls. Depression of cholinesterase activity was noticed in both sexes given doses of 500 or 1000 mg/kg. Female rats fed 500 or 1000 mg/kg diet exhibited an absence of primary follicules and primitive ova and male rats fed 1000 mg/kg diet showed depression of spermatogenesis. Necrotizing arteritis was observed in both sexes at doses of 500 or 1000 mg/kg. However, no treatment-related toxicological changes were reported in rats given 50 or 250 mg/kg diet. The incidences of mammary tumours in female rats were 14, 8, 20, 21, and 25% in groups given 0, 50, 250, 500, and 1000 mg/kg diet, respectively. The time to onset of the appearance of tumours was dose-dependent, being 1.7 years for the controls while at dietary levels of 50, 250, 500, and 1000 mg/kg, the onset occurred after 1.6, 1.8, 1.5, and 1.1 years, respectively (Doull et al., 1962b).

Another long-term toxicity study was reported in which groups each of 25 male and 50 female, 4-week-old, Sprague-Dawley rats were fed trichlorfon at doses of 0, 100, 200, or 400 mg/kg diet for 18 months. Toxicological changes, such as cystic granular alterations of the ovaries and depression of oocytogenesis were seen only in rats fed 400 mg/kg diet. From these 2 studies, it was concluded that trichlorfon given orally to rats may enhance some of the normal aging processes in the reproductive tissues in the females and possibly in the males (Doull et al., 1965).

Groups each comprising 50 male and 50 female, Long-Evans rats, 4 weeks of age, were fed trichlorfon at doses of 50, 250, 500, or 1000 mg/kg diet. A group of 100 male and 100 female rats served as controls. There were neither shortening of survival times nor retarded growth in rats given 1000 mg/kg diet. Depression of cholinesterase activity in both sexes at 1000 mg/kg diet was the only finding related to the treatment. There were no morphological changes considered to be compound-related. All surviving animals were killed after 24 months of treatment. There was no statistically significant difference in the incidence of tumours between treated and control rats (Lorke & Löser, 1966; Grundmann & Hobik, 1966).

A group of 30 male and 35 female albino rats, 10 weeks of age, received 22 mg trichlorfon/kg body weight in saline, by gavage, twice weekly for 90 weeks. A group of 25 male and 26 female rats served as controls. All surviving animals were killed in week 118. Survival time was reduced in the treated group. There were neither biochemical nor morphological changes attributable to the treatment, and no statistically significant differences in the incidence of tumours between treated and control rats (Teichmann et al., 1978).

Groups of 50 male and 50 female Fischer 344 rats, were fed diets containing mean analytical concentrations of 0, 92.2, 273, or 1518 mg trichlorfon/kg feed. Dosages were provided as nominal 0, 100, 300, 1750 mg/kg diet. The top dosage was started as 1000 mg/kg for 27 weeks, changed to 1250 mg/kg for 5 weeks, changed to 1500 mg/kg for 8 weeks, and then changed to 1750 mg/kg for the remaining 65 weeks. Satellite groups of 20 animals per sex served as controls and, at the highest dose level, the animals were treated for one year and then sacrificed to provide interim data. Mortality was unaffected by treatment. Decreased food consumption was slight in females up to 66 weeks and depressed body weight gain occurred in high-dose males. Increased cholesterol levels were observed in males at doses of 300 mg/kg or more while slight anaemia was present in both sexes at 1750 mg/kg. Cholinesterase activity in plasma, red cells, and the brain was significantly reduced in both sexes at 1750 mg/kg. Both liver and kidney weights were increased at 1750 mg/kg in both sexes. Histological changes were not present in the liver; however, chronic nephropathy occurred at the highest dose level. Hyperplasia of the upper small intestine and gastritis occurred at 300 mg/kg and above. A NOEL equal to 4.45 mg/kg body weight for males and 5.82 mg/kg body weight for females was established for the study (Hayes, 1989). Tumorigenicity for this study was not assessed by the Task Group.

8.4.1.3 Dog

Groups each consisting of 2 male and 2 female Beagle dogs were given trichlorfon in the diet at doses of 0, 50, 250, 500, or 1000 mg/kg diet for 12 months. Depression of cholinesterase activity was observed at the 500 and 1000 mg/kg diet levels. Spermatogenesis was inhibited in males given 1000 mg/kg diet (Doull et al., 1962a).

Groups of 4 male and 4 female Beagle dogs were fed dietary trichlorfon at levels of 0, 50, 200, 800, or 3200 mg/kg diet for 4 years. Cholinesterase activity was depressed in dogs of both sexes at doses higher than 200 mg/kg diet. Increased mortality, retarded growth rate, reduced weights of adrenal glands and testes, and impairment of the kidney function were observed at 800 and 3200 mg/kg diet. In addition, cholinergic symptoms, such as tremors, cramps, and salivation were noteworthy at the 3200 mg/kg level. Only one female dog in the latter group survived for 4 years.

Liver injury was detected biochemically in dogs that died during the study (Löser, 1970).

8.4.1.4 Monkey

Groups of 5 male and 5 female Rhesus monkeys (*Macaca mulatta*) were administered technical trichlorfon by gavage at dose levels of 0, 0.2, 1, or 5 mg/kg body weight per day, 6 days per week for 10 years. At the 5 mg/kg level, transient pupillary constriction was seen in 2 animals during the first month, and muscular fasciculations in one. At this dose level, a lowering of the erythrocyte count occurred in both sexes and, towards the end of the study, the body weights were lower in this group. Plasma-, erythrocyte-, and brain-cholinesterase activity was inhibited in the 5 and 1 mg/kg groups, while in the 0.2 mg/kg group inhibition occurred only in erythrocytes in the males. Liver biopsies done during the first 3 years of the study did not reveal any evidence of changed liver morphology in any of the groups. No trichlorfon-related mortality occurred. Complete gross and microscopic examination of the tissues of the treated groups gave a non-neoplastic pathology similar to that in the control group. No significant pathology, including tumorigenicity, related to the administration of trichlorfon was observed in the treated animals, compared with the controls (Griffin, 1988).

8.4.2 Intraperitoneal administration

8.4.2.1 Mouse

A group of 30 male and 30 female AB/Jena strain mice, 8 weeks of age, received 28.2 mg trichlorfon/kg body weight by ip injection, twice weekly, for 75 weeks. A group of 30 male and 30 female control mice were given saline intraperitoneally. All surviving animals were killed in week 80. Inhibition of body weight gain and reduced survival time were noted in the treated group. There was no statistically significant difference in the incidences of tumours between treated and control mice (Teichmann & Hauschild, 1978).

8.4.2.2 *Rat*

In a study by Teichmann et al. (1978), a group of 30 male and 35 female albino rats, 10 weeks of age, received 12 mg trichlorfon/kg body weight intraperitoneally, twice weekly, for 90 weeks, while a group of 25 male and 25 female control rats was given saline. All surviving animals were killed in week 118. Survival time was reduced in the treated group. There was no statistically significant difference in the incidences of tumours between treated and control rats.

8.4.2.3 *Hamster*

Syrian golden hamsters, (23 males and 25 females per group) 7-8 weeks of age, were given 20 mg trichlorfon/kg body weight intraperitoneally, once weekly, for 90 weeks. A group of 22 male and 23 female control hamsters were given saline. All surviving animals were killed in week 100. Inhibition of body weight gain and reduced survival time were noted in the treated group. There was no statistically significant difference in the incidences of tumours between treated and control hamsters (Teichmann & Schmidt, 1978).

8.4.3 *Dermal administration*

8.4.3.1 *Mouse*

A group of 30 male and 30 female AB/Jena strain mice, 8 weeks of age, received 0.25 ml 1% solution of trichlorfon in acetone, dermally, twice weekly, for 75 weeks. A group of 30 male and 30 female mice served as controls. All surviving animals were killed in week 80. Inhibition of body weight gain and reduced survival time were noted in the treated group. There was no statistically significant difference in the incidences of tumours between treated and control mice (Teichmann & Hauschild, 1978).

8.5 Mutagenicity

8.5.1 *DNA methylation*

In vitro studies using chemical agents or isolated nucleic acids with dichlorvos showed that the methylating capability of dichlorvos was less, by a factor of 10-100, than that of strongly genotoxic agents (WHO, 1989). *In vivo* studies using the determination of ^{14}C-N_7-methylguanine in the urine have been used to calculate the *in vivo* methylation capability of dichlorvos for DNA (WHO, 1989) and trichlorfon (Dedek et al., 1976). However, it has been shown that the excretion of $^{14}CH_3$-labelled purines in the urine does not constitute evidence for the methylation of the purines of DNA, because a natural biosynthetic pathway will give rise to urinary methylated purines via the C_1-pool (Wright et al., 1979; WHO, 1989). Consequently, only the measurement of ^{14}C methylated purines in the DNA of organs would provide acceptable results for the evaluation of the *in vivo* methylating capability of alkylating agents (Wright et al., 1979).

Such studies have been performed by Dedek (1981) for trichlorfon with ip administration of 0.48, 0.40, or 0.065 mmol/kg to male mice (strain AB Jena/Halle). The extent of methylation in liver DNA was found to be maximal after 6 h in amounts of 6-8 and 0.8 μmol N_7-MeG/mol guanine for the high and the low dose, respectively, that is 6-8 methylations in the N_7 position per 10^6 guanine bases. However, the alkylation at N_7 of guanine by small groups, such as the methyl group, does not show a good correlation with genotoxic effects.

For obtaining a dose-independent measure of alkylation activity, the covalent binding index may be used, which is defined as:

$$\text{CBI} = \frac{\text{micromol bound per mol of nucleotides}}{\text{millimol administered per kg animal}}$$

For the strong alkylating agent methyl methanesulfonate (MMS), the CBI values for guanine N_7 have been estimated to be between 135 and 556, depending on the route of administration and the time intervals. The corresponding CBI values for trichlorfon were 2.3 to 5.1 (Dedek, 1981; Dedek et al., 1984).

Trichlorfon has a DNA-alkylating property and may react with DNA *in vitro* to cause depurination and excision (Rosenkranz & Rosenkranz, 1972).

8.5.2 *Mutagenicity*

Data on mutagenicity tests *in vitro* as well as *in vivo* have accumulated during the past 20 years. Results indicate that trichlorfon is partly positive and partly negative, depending on the purity of the test material, test system, dosage, or source, and possible effects derived from its degradation products (IARC, 1983). Results are summarized in Table 11.

Trichlorfon induces gene mutation in *S. typhimurium* and *E. coli* (Poole et al., 1977; Carere et al., 1978a; Benigni et al., 1980; Shirasu et al., 1982; Morya et al., 1983) and in *S. cerevisiae* (Riccio et al., 1981; Gilot-Delhalle et al., 1983). It also induces a mitotic crossing over, gene conversion, and mitotic recombination (Waters et al., 1980). The positive results in microorganisms indicate that trichlorfon induces mainly base-pair substitution or mutation in the absence of metabolic activation. Trichlorfon also induces a chlorophyl mutation (Panda & Sharma, 1980) and chromosomal damage in plants (Logvinenko & Morgun, 1978; de Kergommeaux, 1983).

In vitro studies with mammalian cells indicate that trichlorfon induces unscheduled DNA synthesis (UDS) in human epithelial cells (Benigni & Dogliotti, 1980; Aquilina et al., 1984) and in human fibroblasts (Waters et al., 1982). It induces sister chromatid exchanges (SCE) in Chinese hamster ovary (CHO) cells (Chen et al., 1981; Waters et al., 1982), and chromosomal aberrations in CHO (Sasaki et al., 1980; Ishidate et al., 1981) and human lymphocytes (Kurinniy & Pilinskaya, 1977).

Trichlorfon has also been shown to cause cell transformation in C3H1OT1/2 CL8 cells (Waters et al., 1981, 1982), and forward mutations in mouse lymphoma L51784 cells in the absence of metabolic activation (McGregor et al., 1988).

In vivo studies indicate that trichlorfon induces chromosomal aberrations in mouse bone marrow cells (Kurinniy, 1975; Kuzmenko et al., 1980; Ryazanova & Gafurova, 1980; Nehéz et al., 1987). However, negative results have been reported in a bone marrow micronucleus test after intraperitoneal injection of trichlorfon in doses up to 400 mg/kg (Paik & Lee, 1977; Jones et al., 1982; Waters et al., 1982). In the dominant lethal test on mice, trichlorfon was

Table 11. Summary of mutagenicity studies on trichlorfon

Test system		Result	Reference
Microorganisms			
Rec-assay	*P. mirabilis*	+	Adler et al. (1976); Braun et al. (1982)
	S. typhimurium	+	Braun et al. (1982)
	B. subtilis	–	Shirasu et al. (1976)
Spot-test	*E. coli*	–	Nagy et al. (1975)
	S. typhimurium	–	Carere et al. (1978a)
Point mutation	*E. coli*	+	Hanna & Dyer (1975); Batzinger & Bueding (1977); Kawachi et al. (1980); Nagy et al. (1975); Moriya et al. (1983)
	S. typhimurium	+	Poole et al. (1977); Benigni et al. (1980); Carere et al. (1978a); Kawachi et al. (1980); Shirasu et al. (1982)
	A. nidulans	–	Morpurgo et al. (1977); Moriya et al. (1983)
	S. coelicolor	+	Carere et al. (1978a,b); Benigni et al. (1980)
	S. cerevisiae	+	Riccio et al. (1981)
	S. pombe	+	Gilot-Delhalle et al. (1983)
Mitotic crossing over	*A. nidulans*	+	Morpurgo et al. (1977); Benigni et al. (1980)
	S. cerevisiae	+	Riccio et al. (1981); Waters et al. (1982)
Gene conversion	*S. cerevisiae*	+	Riccio et al. (1981); Jones et al. (1982); Waters et al. (1982)
Mitotic recombination	*S. cerevisiae*	+	Poole et al. (1977); Riccio et al. (1981); Simmon (1979); Waters et al. (1982)

Table 11 (continued).

Test system		Result	Reference
Plants			
Chlorophyl gene mutation	*H. vulgare*	+	Panda & Sharma (1980)
Chromosome damage	*H. vulgare*	+	Panda & Sharma (1980)
	Wheat	+	Logvinenko & Morgun (1978)
Clastogenesis	*Vicia faba*	+	Amer & Ali (1983); de Kergommeaux et al. (1983)
Mammalian cells *in vitro*			
UDS	Human epithelial cells	+	Benigni & Dogliotti (1980)
	Human fibroblasts	+	Waters et al. (1982)
SCE	Chinese hamster cells	+	Chen et al. (1981, 1982); Waters et al. (1982)
Mammalian cells *in vitro*			
Chromosome damage	Chinese hamster cells	+	Sasaki et al. (1980); Ishidate et al. (1981)
	Human lymphocytes	+	Kurinniy & Pilinskaya (1977)
Gene mutation	Mouse lymphoma	+	Paik & Lee (1977); Jones et al. (1982); Waters et al. (1982)
Forward mutation assay	Mouse lymphoma cells	+	McGregor et al. (1988)
Drosophila			
Gene mutation	*D. melanogaster*	–	Benes & Sram (1969); Brzheskii (1973); Lamb (1977) Valencia (1977); Waters et al. (1980)
Recessive lethal	*D. melanogaster*	–	Lamb (1977); Waters et al. (1980)

Table 11 (continued).

Mammals			
Micronucleus test	Mouse bone marrow	–	Paik & Lee (1977); Herbold (1979a); Waters et al. (1982); Jones et al. (1982);
Chromosome damage	Mouse bone marrow	–	Degraeve et al. (1981, 1985)
		+	Kurinniy (1975); Nehez et al. (1982, 1987); Degraeve et al. (1981)
	Hamster bone marrow	–	Dzwonkowska & Hübner (1986); Volkner (1987)
Dominant lethal	Mice	–	Arnold et al. (1971); Epstein et al. (1972); Herbold (1979b); Becker & Schoeneich (1980); Degraeve et al. (1981, 1984a); Moutschen-Dahmen (1981)
		+	Schiemann (1975); Dedek et al. (1975)
Chromosome damage	Mouse testes	–	Degraeve et al. (1981, 1984b, 1985)
		+	Bulsiewicz et al. (1976);
		+	Fischer et al. (1977)
Chromosome damage	Human lymphocytes	+	Trinh Van Bao et al. (1974); Kiraly et al. (1979)

reported to induce a significant increase in post implantation losses only after administration of relatively high doses, i.e., 405 mg/kg, as a single dose, or 54 mg/kg, daily, for 3 weeks (Dedek et al., 1975; Fischer et al., 1977). The reproducibility of such effects, however, was not supported by other investigators (Becker & Schöneich, 1980). A short-term study on mice indicated that trichlorfon did not induce any chromosomal damage in either bone marrow or germ cells after treatment with 0.5 mg/litre in the drinking-water, continuously, for 7 weeks (Degraeve et al., 1984).

Cytogenetic studies on lymphocytes obtained from persons suffering from acute intoxication or those occupationally exposed to trichlorfon showed variable increases in the frequency of chromosomal aberrations (Trinh Van Bao et al., 1974; Kiraly et al., 1979).

In conclusion, trichlorfon is mutagenic for microorganisms or mammalian cells in *in vitro* assay systems. However, the data are not consistent, probably because of the purity of the test material and possible effects derived from its degradation products, such as dichlorvos. *In vivo* studies indicate that trichlorfon induces chromosomal damage only at relatively high dose levels. In short-term studies, however, no such effects were found in bone marrow cells or in germ cells.

8.6 Carcinogenicity

All long-term studies available for this evaluation have been described in section 8.4; many of these studies are inadequate as carcinogenicity studies, or the available reports give insufficient detail for an evaluation.

A weak, dose-related increase in the incidence of mammary tumours was reported in female rats fed trichlorfon in the diet (Doull et al., 1962b). However, reports adequate for evaluation did not show any evidence for the carcinogenicity of trichlorfon in rats, mice, or hamsters after oral, intraperitoneal, or skin application.

The carcinogenicity of dichlorvos, the major conversion product of trichlorfon in the mammalian body, has been discussed in WHO (1989) and US NTP (1989) (see section 8.10).

8.7 Teratogenicity and reproductive toxicity

8.7.1 Mouse

A single dose of 360 mg trichlorfon/kg, injected intraperitoneally in 33 AS/Jena mice on the first day of gestation, caused embryotoxicity. Post-implantation losses were increased with 60, 120, 240 mg/kg ip on day 9 of gestation (13-15 mice/group), with 120 or 240 mg/kg ip on days 1-7 (25-30 mice/group), and were more pronounced with 240 mg/kg ip (23 mice) on days 7-14 of gestation. There were no serious malformations (Scheufler, 1975).

Nehéz et al. (1987) showed that 4 consecutive intraperitoneal doses of 51.5 mg trichlorfon/kg body weight administered to AB Jena/Halle mice (12-21 per group) on days 2, 3, 4, and 5, or days 6, 8, 10, and 12 of gestation produced a very weak embryotoxic effect (slightly elevated post-implantation losses, $P < 0.05$), but no teratogenic activity was found.

A dose of 500 or 600 mg trichlorfon/kg body weight, given daily to CD-1 mice by oral gavage on days 10-14 of gestation, produced a reduction in fetal weight and a slightly increased incidence of cleft palate. This malformation was found in 4/67 fetuses from dams given 500 mg/kg, in 7/205 fetuses from dams given 600 mg/kg, and in 3/402 fetuses from control dams (Staples & Goulding, 1979).

When trichlorfon was administered by gavage to CD-1 mice (15-24 per group) on days 7-16 of gestation, at a daily dose of 200, 300, or 400 mg/kg, and to CD rats (15-24 per group) at 50, 100, or 200 mg/kg per day on days 7-19 or 8-20 of gestation, trichlorfon was teratogenic, fetotoxic, and lethal at the two highest dose levels. At the lowest dose level, which was not maternally toxic, there was a significant increase in the number of calcified centres in the forepaws and hindpaws indicating fetotoxicity and a delay in maturation (Courtney et al., 1986).

Clemens & Hartnagel (1986) reviewed this study and suggested that no major or minor birth defects had been demonstrated, and that the embryotoxicity, fetotoxicity, and rib variations in the mouse study occurred at maternally toxic dose levels. The fact that a very small number of fetuses was assessed made conclusions difficult.

Intragastric exposure of male CFW mice (30/group) to 30 mg trichlorfon/kg for 5-260 days resulted in a significant regression of the seminiferous epithelium in the testes after 100 days of treatment. No regeneration of the gonads was observed, 40 days after exposure ceased (Wenda-Rozewicka, 1983).

8.7.2 Rat

A single dose of 80 mg trichlorfon/kg, given to groups of 11 Wistar rats by oral gavage on day 13 of gestation, produced an increased incidence of embryonic death and fetal malformations, such as exencephaly and nonclosing eyelids. When 80 mg trichlorfon/kg was similarly administered on day 9, these effects were not significant. A daily dose of 8 mg/kg during gestation did not produce any teratogenic manifestations (Martson & Voronina, 1976).

When trichlorfon was administered in the diet to groups of 9-26 CD rats on days 6-15 of gestation at a daily intake of 76, 145, 375, 432 or 519 mg/kg body weight, both maternal and fetal body weights were reduced with ingestion of 432 or 519 mg/kg. There was a dose-related increase in the incidence of fetal malformations with ingestion of 145 mg/kg or more. The predominant malformations were exencephaly, meningocoele, hydrocephaly, syndactily, micrognathia, cleft palate, and skeletal system alterations. No adverse effects were found with a dose of 76 mg/kg (Staples et al., 1976).

A daily dose of 480 mg trichlorfon/kg, given to 34 CD rats by gavage on days 6-15 of gestation, produced a high incidence (86%) of fetal malformations, such as generalized oedema, herniation of the brain, hydroencephaly, micrognathia, cleft palate, and skeletal system alterations (Staples & Goulding, 1979).

Groups of 25 naturally inseminated, female Long Evans rats were exposed by gavage to technical trichlorfon at 0, 10, 30, or 100 mg/kg body weight per day from day 6 to day 16 of gestation, and sacrificed on day 20. None of the doses had a lethal effect. Although at 100 mg/kg diarrhoea was caused in some of the animals, embryonic and fetal development were not affected at this dose level (Machemer, 1979a).

Groups of 33 naturally inseminated, female Charles River rats were exposed to technical trichlorfon at 0, 500, 1125, or 2500 mg/kg (equivalent to 0, 45, 102, or 227 mg/kg body weight per day) from day 6 to day 15 of gestation, and sacrificed on day 20. Trichlorfon was maternally toxic at dietary levels of 500, 1125, and 2500 mg/kg. There was no evidence of trichlorfon-related embryotoxicity (increased resorption), fetotoxicity (decreased fetal weight), or teratogenicity (malformations) at exposure levels up to and including 2500 mg/kg. There was an increase in the incidence of delayed ossification and curved, wavy, and/or bulbous ribs at 2500 mg/kg. On the basis of the results of this study, 1125 mg/kg, equivalent to 102 mg/kg body weight per day, is considered the no-observed-effect dose, in terms of reproductive liability (Kowalski et al., 1987).

A 3-generation (2 litters per generation) rat reproduction study with levels of 0, 100, 300, 1000, or 3000 mg trichlorfon/kg in the diet resulted in adverse effects on reproduction at 1000 mg/kg, and above. At 1000 mg/kg, there was evidence of reduced fertility, smaller litters, and reduced body weight of pups. At 3000 mg/kg, the pregnancy rate was markedly decreased and the pups were smaller and lighter in weight with none surviving to the weanling stage. No effects were noted at 300 mg/kg or below. Microscopic examination of tissues from the F_{3b} generation did not indicate any adverse effects (Löser, 1969; Spicer & Urwin, 1971).

8.7.3 Hamster

When 200, 300, or 400 mg trichlorfon/kg body weight was given by gavage to groups of 10-30 female golden hamsters, each day, on days 7-11 of gestation, the 300 and 400 mg/kg doses produced a reduction in maternal food consumption. At 400 mg/kg, there were signs of maternal toxicity and 3 out of 30 animals died; fetal death and malformations (cleft palate, patagium, and fused ribs) were increased. At 300 mg/kg, only one fetus (out of 105) had malformations. A dose of 200 mg/kg body weight did not produce any adverse effects (Staples & Goulding, 1979).

8.7.4 Rabbit

Groups of 15 naturally inseminated, female Himalayan rabbits were exposed by gavage to technical trichlorfon at 0, 5, 15, or 45 mg/kg body weight per day from day 6 to day 18 of gestation and sacrificed on day 29. The average weight gain of the dosed groups was reduced, but doses of 5 and 15 mg/kg were tolerated well. Because of maternal toxic effects, two abortions occurred at 45 mg/kg, but the fetuses delivered in this dose group developed normally. The no-observed-effect level with respect to embryonic development was 15 mg/kg body weight per day. There were no indications that trichlorfon produced any teratogenic effects in this study (Machemer, 1979b).

Groups of 20, artificially inseminated, female American Dutch rabbits were orally exposed to 0, 10, 35, or 110 mg technical trichlorfon/kg body weight per day from day 6 to day 18 of gestation and sacrificed on day 28. The highest dose (110 mg/kg) was not well tolerated and resulted in adverse clinical signs and death, significantly reduced overall body weight gain and food consumption, and significantly inhibited cholinesterase. At 35 mg/kg, cholinesterase was significantly inhibited and one death occurred that was possibly treatment-related. A dose of 10 mg/kg was devoid of overt maternal toxicity, while 110 mg/kg was embryotoxic and fetotoxic, but not teratogenic; 35 mg/kg was a NOEL for developmental toxicity and 10 mg/kg for maternal toxicity (Clemens et al., 1990).

8.7.5 Congenital tremor

Several outbreaks of congenital tremor in piglets have been described in herds in which the sows had been treated with antiparasitic trichlorfon preparations between days 45 and 63 of pregnancy (Kronevi et al., 1975; Dobson, 1977; Bölske et al., 1978; Hansen et al., 1978; Knox et al., 1978). Clinically, the disease was characterized by ataxia and tremor and a pronounced hypoplasia of the cerebellum was found, as well as a reduction in the size of the spinal cord.

This disease was reproduced experimentally. Four sows were dosed with Neguvon Vet at 60 mg/kg body weight, mixed in the morning feed on day 55 and on day 70 of pregnancy. All 40 piglets born alive showed ataxia and tremor, and, at autopsy, hypoplasia of the cerebellum. In 97 control litters, none of the 892 live-born piglets showed nervous signs (Knox et al., 1978). Similar experimental results were obtained following exposure of pigs to multiple oral doses of 50-75 mg trichlorfon/kg between approximately 45 and 63 days after conception (Pope et al., 1986; Berge et al., 1987a; Rasmussen et al., 1978). A similar, but less severe effect resulted from the post-natal exposure of piglets from week 3 to week 6 to 50 mg/kg body weight per day. Recovery of animals exposed prenatally was slow; 35 days after birth they had not reached control values for cerebral and cerebellar weight. There was still regional loss of Purkinje cells in the cerebellum (Berge et al., 1987b).

Ten pregnant, white guinea-pigs were given 6 doses of 100 mg trichlorfon/kg body weight by gavage on days 36, 37, 38, 51, 52, and 53 of pregnancy; 7 additional animals served as controls. The pups developed trembling and locomotor disturbances. Post-mortem examination of the pups revealed significantly decreased weights of the total brain and the cerebellum, compared with controls. There was also a significant weight reduction, particularly of the medulla oblongata, but also of the hippocampus, the thalamus, and the colliculi. Histological examination of the cerebellum revealed reduction of the external granular layer, and the molecular layer, together with a regional absence of Purkinje cells. The activities of the neurotransmitter enzymes cholineacetyltransferase and glutamate decarboxylase in the cerebellum were reduced compared with the control values (Berge et al., 1986). Pregnant, albino guinea-pigs were given radiolabelled trichlorfon on days 37 or 52 of pregnancy and examined by whole body autoradiography 15, 30, and 45 min after administration. Trichlorfon had not accumulated in the fetal guinea-pig brain (Berge & Nafstad, 1986).

8.8 Neurotoxicity

Olajos et al. (1979) reported that the administration of a divided dose of 300 mg/kg to hens (200 + 100 mg/kg given subcutaneously, 3 days apart) resulted in levels of neurotoxic esterase (NTE) inhibition (46-68% at 24 h) approaching the 70% level that has been correlated with the development of organophosphorus- ester-induced delayed neurotoxicity (OPIDN), and moderate clinical signs (ataxia) resembling the early stages of OPIDN. Shiraishi et al. (1983) produced a peripheral neuropathy in a single monkey (1 out of 1) with a single dose of 250 mg/kg.

Based on a review of the literature on trichlorfon and dichlorvos (both animal studies and cases of human poisoning), Johnson (1981, 1990), Caroldi & Lotti (1981), and WHO (1989) concluded that only doses that exceed the lethal dose are likely to result in a level of NTE inhibition at which OPIDN would be expected. Johnson summarized reports of neurotoxicity studies on trichlorfon in hens as follows: The acute maximum tolerated cholinergic dose (200 mg/kg subcutaneously) produced no marked neuropathy in hens; however, moderate neuropathy was seen when a further dose of 100 mg/kg was given subcutaneously, 3 days later. Histological signs of severe degeneration were seen in the sciatic nerve and spinal cord of the ataxic bird at autopsy after 3 weeks. Slight changes were reported in sections of the brain stem of the birds given 200 mg/kg, orally, or 100 mg/kg, subcutaneously (Olajos et al., 1979). But these did not appear to be entirely typical of organophosphorus neuropathy and no lesions were reported for the spinal cord or sciatic nerve. Inhibition of NTE in the spinal cord was only measured in later studies (Hierons & Johnson, 1978) and lagged markedly behind that in the brain.

The ability of trichlorfon to induce delayed neurotoxicity was assessed in adult White Leghorn hens, administered single subcutaneous doses of 100 or 300 mg/kg, and assessed for visible signs of neurotoxicity 24 h after treatment, prior to killing and collection of samples of brain and spinal (cervical, thoracic) cord for the measurement of AChE and NTE activities. In short-term studies, hens received trichlorfon (100 mg/kg) every 72 h for a total of 6 doses. Three days after the terminal dose, the hens were killed and the brains, spinal cords, and distal sciatic nerves were removed for enzymatic and histological examination. While trichlorfon markedly inhibited tissue AChE, no reduction in NTE was detected and no overt signs of neurotoxicity were observed. In the short-term studies, trichlorfon did not cause any obvious neurotoxicity, an observation supported by minimal changes in the spinal cord and sciatic nerve morphology, no impairment of walking ability, and no inhibition of the brain and spinal cord NTE (Slott & Ecobichon, 1984).

A number of other reports indicate that trichlorfon is either not neurotoxic, or produces a neurotoxic effect that is distinct from OPIDN. In addition to the Slott & Ecobichon study, several short-term dosing regimens that resulted in severe cholinergic toxicity by either the oral (Olajos et al., 1979) or dermal (Francis et al., 1985) route did not result in neuropathy. Oral doses of 100 mg trichlorfon/kg were also reported not to result in significant NTE inhibition (Olajos et al., 1979; Olajos & Rosenblum, 1981). Finally, rats, which are much less sensitive to agents that cause delayed neurotoxicity, exhibited electrophysiological signs of neurotoxicity without accompanying histological changes when given oral doses of 30 mg/kg for 3 weeks (Lehotzky, 1982) or ip injections of trichlorfon at 200 mg/kg per day for 5-15 days (Averbook & Anderson, 1983).

Other adverse neurobehavioural effects that have been observed may be due to acetylcholinesterase inhibition. Dési (1983) exposed adult CFY rats (10 males and 10 females per group) at levels of 16 and 32 mg/kg for 3 months. The lower dose resulted in increased high-frequency EEC activity and enhanced central excitability, and the higher dose in increased low-frequency EEG activity and a significant overall increase in EEG activity, as well as indications of depressed cortical excitability. In animals treated orally with trichlorfon at 30 mg/kg per day, increased locomotor activity in the open field and decreased rotorod performance were observed transiently. While the animals were able to acquire the conditioned escape reflex, latency of the escape responses in the conditioned escape reflex was markedly increased (Lehotzky, 1982).

8.9 Immunological studies

Exposure of female mice (BALB/cByJ & C57BL/6J strain; 4 per group) to 175 mg trichlorfon/100 ml drinking-water for 14 days had no effect on immune function, measured by response to influenza virus (Reiss et al., 1987). The dose used was considered to be effective for prophylactic treatment against helminthic infestation.

8.10 Toxicity of dichlorvos

The major transformation product of trichlorfon in mammals, including human beings, is dichlorvos, which is at least 100 times more active as a cholinesterase inhibitor than trichlorfon (Hofer, 1981). An evaluation of the health and environmental hazards of dichlorvos can be found in WHO (1989). For completeness sake, however, the summary on effects on experimental animals and *in vitro* test systems from this publication is reproduced below.

"Dichlorvos is moderately to highly toxic when administered in single doses to a variety of animals species by several routes. It directly inhibits acetylcholinesterase (AChE) activity in the nervous system and in other tissues. Maximum inhibition generally occurs within 1 h, and is followed by rapid recovery. The oral LD_{50} for the rat is 30-110 mg/kg body weight, depending on the solvent used. The hazard classification of dichlorvos by WHO is based on an oral LD_{50} for the rat of 56 mg/kg body weight. The signs of intoxication are typical of organophosphorus poisoning, i.e., salivation, lachrymation, diarrhoea, tremors, and terminal convulsions, with death occurring from respiratory failure. The signs of intoxication are usually apparent shortly after dosing, and, at lethal doses, death occurs within 1 h. Survivors recover completely within 24 h.

Potentiation is slight when dichlorvos is given orally in combination with other organophosphates, but in combination with malathion it is marked.

In short-term toxicity studies on the mouse, rat, dog, pig, and monkey, inhibition of plasma, red blood cell, and brain ChE are the most important signs of toxicity. After oral administration, a dose of approximately 0.5 mg/kg body weight (range, 0.3-0.7 mg/kg) did not produce ChE inhibition. In a 2-year study on dogs, ChE inhibition was noted at 3.2 mg/kg body weight or more.

Flea collar dermatitis has been described in dogs and cats wearing dichlorvos-impregnated PVC flea collars. This was a primary irritant contact dermatitis that may have been caused by dichlorvos.

Many short-term, inhalation studies on different animal species have been carried out. Air concentrations in the range of 0.2-1 mg/m^3 do not affect ChE activity significantly. Other effects, such as growth inhibition and increase in liver weight, have been reported at dose levels at least 10-20 times higher.

It is possible to produce clinical neuropathy in hens, but the doses of dichlorvos required are far in excess of the LD_{50}. The effects are associated with high inhibition of neurotoxic esterase (NTE) in the brain and spinal cord. In the rat, however, neuropathic changes in the white matter of the brain have been reported following repeated daily oral application of an LD_{50} dose.

Immune suppression has been reported in rabbits. At present, no evaluation as to the relevance for human beings can be given; more attention to this aspect is needed.

In a long-term study, rats fed dichlorvos in the diet for 2 years showed no signs of intoxication. Hepatocellular fatty vacuolization of the liver and ChE inhibition were significant at the two highest dose levels (2.5 and 12.5 mg/kg body weight).

In a carefully conducted, long-term, inhalation study on rats with whole body exposure (23 h/day, for 2 years), results were comparable with those seen in the oral study. No effects were seen at 0.05 mg/m^3, inhibition of ChE activity took place at 0.48 mg/m^3 or more.

In several reproduction studies on rats and domestic animals, no effects were seen on reproduction, and there was no embryotoxicity at dose levels that did not cause maternal toxicity. At toxic doses, dichlorvos may cause reversible disturbances of spermatogenesis in mice and rats. It was not teratogenic in several studies carried out on rats and rabbits.

Dichlorvos is an alkylating agent and binds *in vitro* to bacterial and mammalian nucleic acids. It is mutagenic in a number of microbial systems, but there is no evidence of mutagenicity in intact mammals, where it is rapidly degraded by esterases in blood and other tissues.

Dichlorvos carcinogenicity has been investigated in mice (oral studies) and rats (oral and inhalation studies). The dose levels used in 2-year, oral studies were up to 800 mg/litre drinking-water or 600 mg/kg diet for mice, and up to 280 mg/litre drinking-water or 234 mg/kg diet for rats. In a rat inhalation study, dichlorvos concentrations in air of up to 4.7 mg/m^3 were tested for 2 years. No statistically significant increase in tumour incidence was found. In two recent carcinogenicity studies on mice and rats, dichlorvos was administered by intubation at dose levels between 10 and 40 mg/kg body weight (mice) and 4 and 8 mg/kg body weight (rat) for up to 2 years. Only preliminary information has been provided. The evidence for carcinogenicity in these new studies is difficult to interpret at this time. Only when complete and final reports become available will it be possible to draw more definitive conclusions.[a]

From acute and short-term studies, it is clear that the metabolites of dichlorvos are all less toxic than the parent compound. Only dichloroacetaldehyde was positive in a few mutagenicity tests."

8.11 Mechanism of toxicity - mode of action

While trichlorfon itself is not a potent anticholinesterase agent, the inhibiting activity of this chemical is attributed to the transformation product dichlorvos. The slow conversion of trichlorfon to dichlorvos results in the inhibition of both central and peripheral cholinergic nerve acetylcholinesterase, with the accumulation of the neurotransmitter, acetylcholine, at nerve endings, and the generation of characteristic signs and symptoms of toxicity. A full description of the mechanism of action of organophosphorus ester insecticides can be found in Environmental Health Criteria No. 63: *Organophosphorus insecticides - a general introduction* (WHO, 1986), and that of dichlorvos in Environmental Health Criteria No. 79: Dichlorvos (WHO, 1989). The muscarinic, nicotinic, and the central nervous system-induced signs and symptoms observed in humans have been described extensively (Ecobichon et al., 1977; Hayes, 1982; Hayes & Laws, 1991).

Transformation of trichlorfon to dichlorvos *in vivo* was studied in relation to its effects on the cholinesterase activity, acetylcholine

---

[a] The US-NTP Peer Review Panel reviewed these studies and came to the following conclusions: "Under the conditions of these 2-year gavage studies, there was some evidence of carcinogenic activity of dichlorvos for male F344/N rats, as shown by increased incidences of adenomas of the exocrine pancreas and mononuclear cell leukemia. There was equivocal evidence of carcinogenic activity of dichlorvos for female F344/N rats, as shown by increased incidences of adenomas of the exocrine pancreas and mammary gland fibroadenomas. There was some evidence of carcinogenic activity of dichlorvos for male B6C3F1 mice and clear evidence for female B6C3F1 mice, as shown by increased incidences of forestomach squamous cell papillomas." (US-NTP, 1989).
In a recent evaluation of current data, IARC (in press) concluded that there is sufficient evidence for the carcinogenicity of dichlorvos in experimental animals, but that there is inadequate evidence for the carcinogenicity of dichlorvos in humans.

content, and acetylcholine-turnover in the mouse brain. An ip injection of 10 mg dichlorvos/kg caused toxic signs, such as salivation, diarrhoea and, in some cases, difficulties in breathing, which were clearly recognized about 15 min after administration and disappeared almost completely towards the end of 60 min. After an ip injection of 125 mg trichlorfon/kg, the above mentioned signs were most intense at around 30 min; and almost complete recovery was observed towards the end of 2 h. The cholinesterase activity and acetylcholine levels reached their minimum and maximum, respectively, at 15 min after the injection of dichlorvos and about 45 min after the injection of trichlorfon. The delayed decrease in acetylcholine turnover following to ip injection of trichlorfon was also demonstrated by measuring the acetylcholine-synthesizing rate in the brain following intravenous injection of $^{2}H_{6}$-choline compared with dichlorvos pretreatment. The level of dichlorvos in the brain of mice administered trichlorfon ip reached its maximum a few minutes after the maximal level of trichlorfon itself; both compounds decreased over similar curves during a 120-min period (Nordgren et al., 1978).

Thirty minutes after intraventricular injection of trichlorfon (2.5 mg) in the rat, the activity of the cholinesterase decreased to 20% in the hippocampus; 22% in the medulla; 50% in the cerebellum; 58% in the striatum, and 72% in the cortex. Levels of acetylcholine reached a maximum at 45 min in the hippocampus and cortex, and peaked in the striatum at 60 min. The greatest increases were seen in the hippocampus and cortex with 60 and 55%, respectively (Hallak & Giacobini, 1987).

The administration of 80 mg trichlorfon/kg im to male Sprague-Dawley rats was found to produce an increase in acetylcholine levels, which peaked at about 170% of control levels, 30 min after exposure (Hallak & Giacobini, 1989). Acetylcholine levels returned to normal within 120 min of exposure. A second dose at 120 min resulted in a second surge in the acetylcholine levels.

9. EFFECTS ON HUMAN BEINGS

Trichlorfon is one of the organophosphorus compounds for which not only acutely toxic effects have been described, but also delayed neurotoxicity in humans (WHO, 1986).

In addition to the reports describing cases of human poisoning, there is wide experience concerning the therapeutic use of trichlorfon and the side-effects arising from this use.

9.1 Acute poisoning - poisoning incidents

Several hundred cases of acute trichlorfon poisoning, some of them lethal, have been described in the literature. These were either accidental, intentional (suicide), or due to gross neglect of prescriptions or safety precautions. A critical detailed review of these cases is given by Johnson (1981) and Hayes (1982).

In all cases, the onset of poisoning was rapid, early signs and symptoms being exhaustion, headache, weakness, confusion, vomiting, abdominal pain, excessive sweating, and salivation. The pupils are small. Difficulty in breathing may be experienced, because of either congestion of the lungs or weakness of the respiratory muscles. In severe cases of poisoning, muscle spasms, unconsciousness, and convulsions may develop and death may result from respiratory failure.

In the case of trichlorfon, unconsciousness is disproportionately common and prolonged and the incidence of mental disturbances is high; moreover polyneuropathy has been found at a later stage, in approximately 21% of cases (Hayes, 1982). However, after reviewing the literature, Johnson (1981; 1990) concluded that only doses of trichlorfon that exceed the lethal dose, and where the victim survived because of treatment, are likely to result in a level of NTE inhibition at which delayed neurotoxicity would be expected.

The onset of polyneuropathy has occurred as early as 3 days after ingestion and as late as 26 days (Hayes, 1982), the majority of cases following recovery from the acute effects. The clinical, electrophysiological, and histopathological features of the neuropathy were similar to the syndrome resulting from TOCP exposure (Hierons & Johnson, 1978; Shiraishi et al., 1983; Vasilescu et al., 1984; Niedziella et al., 1985). Hayes (1982) discusses the possibility that the polyneuropathy could be caused by other chemical compounds, present as impurities in the technical product or formulation. Johnson (1981) mentions higher alkyl analogs as an example. No confirmation for this hypothesis can be found.

In a case of trichlorfon poisoning, a 21-year-old female attempted suicide by drinking about 50 ml of a 50% formulation of trichlorfon. She lost consciousness and recovered after 8 h. Two weeks after ingestion, the patient developed a tingling sensation in all extremities followed by weakness in the lower limbs and knees, characterized as motor dominant polyneuropathy (Shiraishi et al., 1977).

Progressive neuropathy developed 2-8 weeks after acute poisoning (i.e., unconsciousness for 16 h) in a 20-year-old man who had taken orally a handful of granular solid formulation (trichlorfon content: 80%). The clinical symptoms were typical of the delayed neuropathy that is caused by organophosphates, such as tri-*o*-cresyl-phosphate, with normal conduction velocity in surviving motor nerve fibres as an electrophysiological finding. However, a single dose of the above granular solid sample did not produce acute delayed neurotoxicity in hens (Hierons & Johnson, 1978).

A 42-year-old man was in deep coma after ingestion of 100-200 ml Soldep (25% trichlorfon) and had to be artificially ventilated for 37 days. Plasma cholinesterase activity was significantly decreased. Three weeks after ingestion, there was severe weakness of the lower limbs. The EMG (at 40 and 70 days, 4,6,9, and 14 months) indicated denervation in the lower extremities and peripheral motorneuron lesions in the upper extremities. Twenty-one months after poisoning, there was a slow improvement in mobility and the patient was able to walk by himself for a short distance (Bátora et al., 1988).

Akimov & Kolesnichenko (1985) examined the morphological changes in the nervous system of 14 patients who had died from acute chlorophos poisoning. They found congested blood vessels with perivascular oedema and degeneration of the collagenous- and elastic fibres of the vascular walls. Diffuse cellular changes, such as swelling and ischaemic changes, were found in the brain, spinal cord, and vegetative ganglia. There was a moderate destruction of the myelin sheaths in the lateral columns of the spinal cord and the brain peduncles, and there were structural changes in the axons of the peripheral nerves.

Csik et al. (1986) observed 70 cases of trichlorfon poisoning (mainly suicide attempts) between 1971 and 1983. Twenty-five of them were re-examined in 1984. Nine of these (36%) had severe residual signs of delayed polyneuropathy, mainly of the distal motor type. In one case, signs of CNS lesions had persisted. Four had had complaints (paraesthesia, weakness of hands) 2-3 months after poisoning, but were healthy at the time of re-examination.

9.2 Therapeutic use of trichlorfon

Under the name metrifonate, trichlorfon is used to treat infection by *Schistosomiasis haematobium* in humans (WHO, 1985). Metrifonate has, by now, been given to millions of patients in the tropics in the treatment of schistosomiasis.

Following a dose of 7-12 mg/kg, severe cholinergic symptoms are rare in spite of almost complete inhibition of plasma cholinesterase and 40-60% inhibition of erythrocyte acetylcholinesterase (Nordgren et al., 1981; Davis, 1986). However, trials in which several doses were administered on either the same day or one day apart resulted in abdominal colic, nausea, salivation, dizziness, and headache, which precluded further treatment (Aden-Abdi et al., 1987), and the subject-reported incidence of one or more of these effects after a single dose of 10 mg/kg (46%) was generally higher than in subjects given a vitamin placebo (34%) (Wilkins & Moore, 1987). There is one report of a possible human birth defect resulting from metrifonate treatment (Monson & Alexander, 1984).

In another report on 6000 people, mostly in South Africa and South America, who had been treated with trichlorfon for a few years to control various intestinal and body parasites, the dosages varied from 7.5 up to 70 mg/kg. The dose of 7.5 mg/kg, given 2-4 times at two-week intervals, caused cholinesterase inhibition, weakness, nausea, diarrhoea, and abdominal pain. Higher doses (24 mg/kg) caused more severe symptoms including tachycardia, salivation, colic pain, vomiting, nausea, fatigue, tremors, and sweating. The effects were not cumulative and recovery in all cases was rapid. In a few human cases, an indication was given that spermatogenesis (size and shape of sperm) and sperm mobility might be affected (Wegner, 1970).

In a large-scale programme in rural villages in Somalia, metrifonate was given at a current dosage regimen of 3 single doses of 7.5 mg/kg each, on three separate days at intervals of 2 weeks (Aden Abdi & Gustafsson, 1989). In a large number of cases, the results were not satisfactory, due to poor patient compliance with the treatment regimen. In an attempt to simplify this regimen, 5 mg/kg, given thrice during one day, gave the best results as regards safety and the cure rates were comparable with those with the standard regimen (Aden Abdi, 1990).

In a clinical trial on 20 patients with Alzheimer disease, Becker et al. (1990) gave single oral doses of 2.5, 5, 7.5, or 15 mg metrifonate/kg per week, for 1-3 months. A statistically significant improvement was obtained with the 5 mg/kg per week dose level. A 60% depression in red cell ChE and 80% depression in plasma ChE were accompanied by only minor side effects (nausea, vomiting, and/or diarrhoea); there were no effects at 2.5 mg/kg, 5 patients were affected at 5 mg/kg, 9 at 7.5 mg/kg, and 13 at 15 mg/kg per week.

9.3 Occupational exposures

Few cases of occupational poisoning by trichlorfon have been reported. See section 5.3 for occupational exposures.

Occupational exposure to trichlorfon at a factory where air concentrations exceeded 0.5 mg/m^3, but where skin contamination also occurred, resulted in decreased plasma cholinesterase levels and changes in EEG patterns; particularly slow and paroxysmal waves were observed (Lu et al., 1984; Hu et al., 1986). Both the biochemical and electrophysiological indices returned to normal after exposure ceased.

Although trichlorfon has been widely used for many years, no cases of skin sensitization have been reported (Mihail, 1986b).

9.4 Treatment of acute trichlorfon poisoning

The advice on the treatment of organophosphate poisoning from EHC 63: Organophosphorus insecticides - a general introduction, has been reproduced in Annex I.

10. PREVIOUS EVALUATIONS BY INTERNATIONAL BODIES

Trichlorfon was evaluated by the Joint FAO/WHO Expert Committee on Pesticide Residues (JMPR) in 1971, 1975, and 1978 (FAO/WHO, 1972, 1976, 1979). In 1978, the JMPR established an Acceptable Daily Intake (ADI) for man of 0-0.01 mg/kg body weight, based on the fact that the following levels cause no toxicological effects:

Rat: 50 mg/kg in the diet equivalent to 2.5 mg/kg body weight.
Dog: 50 mg/kg in the diet equivalent to 1.25 mg/kg body weight.

In 1986, the FAO/WHO CODEX Committee advised a range of maximum residue limits (MRLs) for specified food commodities (FAO/WHO, 1986). These ranged from 0.05 to 2 mg/kg product.

Trichlorfon was evaluated by an IARC Working Group in 1983. There were no data on its carcinogenicity in humans and the evidence of carcinogenicity in experimental animals was inadequate. Trichlorfon was classified in Group 3, i.e., cannot be classified as to its carcinogenicity to humans (IARC, 1983, 1987).

WHO classified technical trichlorfon as "slightly hazardous" (Class III) (WHO, 1990). A data sheet on trichlorfon (No. 27) has been published by the WHO (WHO/FAO, 1977).

REFERENCES

ABBASOV, T.A. (1972) [Residues of organophosphorus insecticides in clover and potato plants.] *Khim. Sel'sk. Khoz.*, **10**: 597-598 (in Russian).

ABDEL-KADER, M.I.A., MOUBASHER, A.H., & ABDEL-HAFEZ, S.I. (1978) Selective effects of five pesticides on soil and cotton-rhizosphere and -rhizoplane fungus flora. *Mycopathologia*, **66**: 117-123.

ABDELWAHAB, A.M., KHALIL, F.M., & HUSSEIN, M.H. (1973) Toxicity of insecticides to honey bees in laboratory and field. *Bull. Entomo. Soc. Egypt, Econ. Ser.*, **VII**: 83-89.

ADEN ABDI, Y. (1990) A rational approach to the treatment of *Schistosoma haematobium* infection with metrifonate - clinical and pharmacological studies, Stockholm, Karolinska Institute, Department of Clinical Pharmacology (Thesis).

ADEN ABDI, Y. & GUSTAFSSON, L.L. (1989) Poor patient compliance reduces the efficacy of metrifonate treatment of *Schistosoma haematobium* in Somalia. *Eur. J. clin. Pharmacol.*, **36**: 161-164.

ADEN ABDI, Y., GUSTAFSSON, L.L., & ELMI, S.A. (1987) A simplified dosage schedule of metrifonate in the treatment of *Schistosoma haematobium* infection in Somalia. *Eur. J. clin. Pharmacol.*, **32**: 437- 441.

ADLER, B., BRAUN, R., SCHÖNEICH, J., & BÖHME, H. (1976) Repair-defective mutants of *Proteus mirabilis* as a prescreening system for the detection of potential carcinogens. *Biol. Zentralbl.*, **95**: 463- 469.

AHMAD, Z. & JOHANSEN, C. (1973) Selective toxicity of carbophenothion and trichlorfon to the honey bee and the alfalfa leafcutting bee. *Environ. Entomol.*, **2**: 27-30.

AKHTAR, M.H. (1982) Fate of trichlorfon in buffer and soluble fraction (105 000g) from cow and chicken liver homogenates. *J. agric. food Chem.*, **30**: 551-554.

AKIMOV, G.A. & KOLESNICHENKO, I.P. (1985) [Morphological changes in the nervous system in acute peroral chlorophos poisoning.] *Arkh. Patol.*, **47**(1): 44-51 (in Russian).

AKSNES, G. & YÜKSEKISIK, N. (1974) Kinetic study of the alkaline hydrolysis of 2,2,2-trichloro-1-hydroxyethyl, dimethyl phosphonate, Dipterex, and its ethyl analog. *Phosphorus*, **4**: 33-38.

AMBRUS, A., HARGITAI, E., KAROLY, G., FULOP, A., & LANTOS, J. (1981) General method for determination of pesticide residues in samples of plant origin, soil, and water. II. Thin layer chromatographic determination. *J. Assoc. Off. Anal. Chem.*, **64**: 743-748.

AMENO, K., FUKE, C., AMENO, S., KIRIU, T., & IJIRI, I. (1989) A rapid and sensitive quantitation of dipterex in serum by solid-phase extraction and gas chromatography with flame thermionic detection. *J. anal. Toxicol.*, **13**: 150-151.

AMER, S.M. & ALI, E.M. (1983) Cytological effects of pesticides. XIV. Effect of the insecticide Dipterex "trichlorfon" on *Vicia faba* plant. *Cytologia*, **48**: 761-770.

ANDREU-MOLINER, E.S., ALMAR, M.M., LEGARRA, I., & NUNEZ, A. (1986) Toxicity of some rice-field pesticides to the crayfish *P. Clarkii* under laboratory and field conditions in Lake Albuferra (Spain). *J. environ. Sci. Health*, **B 21**: 529-537.

ANON (1978a) Information on trichlorfon residues surveillance available to FAO/WHO from Hungary.

ANON (1978b) Information on trichlorfon residues available to FAO/WHO from Finland.

ANON (1978c) Information on trichlorfon residues available to FAO/WHO from Netherlands.

ANTOINE, O. & MEES, G. (1971) Test de routine pour la détermination des insecticides organo-phosphorés par la chromatographie en couche mince. *J. Chromatogr.*, **58**: 247-256.

AQUILINA, G., BENIGNI, R., BIGNAMI, M., CALCAGNILE, A., DOGLIOTTI, E., FALCONE, E., & CARERE, A. (1984) Genotoxic activity of dichlorvos, trichlorfon, and dichloroacetaldehyde. *Pestic. Sci.*, **15**: 439-442.

ARNOLD, D., KEPLINGER, M.L., FANCHER, O.E. & CALANDRA, J.C. (1971) *Mutagenic study with Dylox in Albino mice*. Industrial Biotest Laboratories (Unpublished report submitted to WHO by Farbenfabriken Bayer A.G., Germany).

ARTHUR, B.W. & CASIDA, J.E. (1957) Metabolism and selectivity of *O,O*-dimethyl 2,2,2-trichloro-1-hydroxyethylphosphonate and its acetyl and vinyl derivatives. *J. agric. food Chem.*, **5**: 186-192.

AVERBOOK, B.J. & ANDERSON, R.J. (1983) Electrophysiological changes associated with chronic administration of organophosphates. *Arch. Toxicol.*, **52**: 167-172.

BAIDA, T.A. (1970) [Soil pollution by organophosphorus pesticides.] *Kazakstana*, **30**: 72 (in Russian).

BAIDA, T.A. (1975) [Dynamics and metabolism of chlorophos in cabbage and onion plants.] *Khim. Sel'sk Khoz.*, **13**: 67-68 (in Russian).

BARCELO, D. (1988) Application of thermospray liquid chromatography/ mass spectrometry for determination of organophosphorus pesticides and trialkyl and triaryl phosphates. *Biomed. environ. mass Spectrom.*, **17**: 363-369.

BARCELO, D., MARIS, F.A., GEERDINK, R.B., FREI, R.W., DE JONG, G.J., & BRINKMAN, U.A.T. (1987) Comparison between positive, negative and chloride-enhanced negative chemical ionization of organophosphorus pesticides in on-line liquid chromatography-mass spectrometry. *J. Chromatogr.*, **394**: 65-67.

BARTHEL, W.F., GIANG, P.A., & HALL, S.A. (1954) Dialkyl-α-hydroxyphosphonates derived from chloral. *J. Am. Chem. Soc.*, **76**: 4186-4187.

BATORA, I., KUKUMBERG, P., KUCHAR, M., & KOUTUN, J. (1988) [Delayed neurotoxic effect of Soldep (trichlorfon) after acute poisoning.] *Prac. Lèk.*, **40**: 172-174 (in Slovak).

BATTELLE (1982) *Pesticide programme of research and market planning. Part II. Insecticides,* Geneva, Battelle Institute, 40 pp.

BATTELLE (1984) Trichlorfon. In: *World pesticide programme. Insecticides II. World summary: USA, Canada, Argentina, Brazil, Colombia, Mexico, Central America*, Geneva, Battelle Research Centres, pp. 16, 26, 30, 34.

BATTELLE (1987) Trichlorfon. In: *World pesticide programme. Insecticides III. Summary: USA, Mexico, Brazil*, Geneva, Battelle Research Centres, Vol. 1, pp. 6-8, 11, 14, 16-17, 27.

BATZINGER, R.P. & BUEDING, E. (1977) Mutagenic activities *in vitro* and *in vivo* of five antischistosomal compounds. *J. Pharmacol. exp. Ther.*, **200**: 1-9.

BECKER, K. & SCHÖNEICH, J. (1980) Dominant lethal test with trichlorphon in male mice. *Mutat. Res.*, **74**: 224, (Meeting abstract).

BECKER, R.E., COLLIVER, J., ELBLE, R., FELDMAN, E., GIACOBINI, E., KUMAR, V., MARKWELL, S., MORIEARTY, P., PARKS, R., SHILLCUT, S.D., UNNI, L., VICARI, S., WOMACK, C., & ZEC, R.F. (1990) Effects of metrifonate, a long-acting cholinesterase inhibitor in Alzheimer Disease: report of an open trial. *Drug Dev. Res.*, **19**: 425-434.

BEDFORD, C.T. & ROBINSON, J. (1972) The alkylating properties of organophosphates. *Xenobiotica*, **2**: 307-337.

BELLO, T.R., AMBORSKI, G.F., & TORBERT, B.J. (1974) Effects of organic phosphorus anthelmintics on blood cholinesterase values in horses and ponies. *Am. J. vet. Res.*, **35**: 73-78.

BENES, V. & CERNA, V. (1970) Contribution to the toxicological evaluation of fenitrothion (*O*,*O*-dimethyl-*O*-/3-methyl-4-nitrophenyl/thio-phosphate)and its residues. In: Halas et al., ed. *Proceedings of pesticide Symposia Inter-American Conferences on Toxicology and Occupational Medicine, Miami.*

BENES, V. & SRAM, R. (1969) Mutagenic activity of some pesticides in *Drosophila melanogaster. Ind. Med. Surg.*, **38**: 442-444.

BENIGNI, R. & DOGLIOTTI, E. (1980) UDS studies on selected environmental chemicals. *Mutat. Res.*, **74**: 217, 248-249 (Meeting abstract).

BENIGNI, R., BIGNAMI, M., CARERE, A., DOGLIOTTI, E., NOVELLETO, A., & PRINCIPE, R. (1980) Comparative mutational studies with dichlorvos, trichlorfon and dichloroacetaldehyde. *Toxicol. Lett.*, 1(Spec. Issue): 250 (Meeting abstract).

BENNEWITZ, R. & FOTH, G. (1967) [Chemical behavior and analytical determination of trichlorfon, dichlorvos and tribufon.] *Fresenius Z. anal. Chem.*, **229**: 110-117 (in German).

BERGE, G.N. & NAFSTAD, I. (1986) Distribution and placental transfer of trichlorfon in guinea-pigs. *Arch. Toxicol.*, **59**: 26-29.

BERGE, G.N., NAFSTAD, I., & FONNUM, F. (1986) Prenatal effects of trichlorfon on the guinea-pig brain. *Arch. Toxicol.*, **59**: 30-35.

BERGE, G.N., FONNUM, F., & BRODAL, P. (1987a) Neurotoxic effects of prenatal trichlorfon administration in pigs. *Acta vet. Scand.*, **28**: 321-332.

BERGE, G.N., FONNUM, F., SOLI, N.E., & SOGNEN, E. (1987b) Neurotoxicological examination of the piglet brain after prenatal and postnatal exposure to trichlorfon. *Acta vet. Scand.*, **28**: 313-320.

BETOWSKI, L.D. & JONES, T.L. (1988) Analysis of organophosphorus pesticide samples by high-performance liquid chromatography/mass spectrometry and high-performance liquid chromatography/mass spectrometry/mass spectrometry. *Environ. Sci. Technol.*, **22**: 1430-1434.

BOLOTNYI, A.V., PISMENNAYA, M.V., & AKORONKO, S.A. (1978) [Transformation of the organophosphorus pesticides anthiophos and trichlorfon in the environment.] *Gig. i Sanit.*, **1978**(5): 28-31 (in Russian).

BOLSKE, G., KRONEVI, T., & LINDGREN, N.O. (1978) Congenital tremor in pigs in Sweden. *Nord. vet. Med.*, **30**: 534-537.

BOND, G.P. (1986) *Primary dermal irritation of technical trichlorfon (Dylox®) in albino rabbits*, Metcalf, USA, Mobay Corporation, (Proprietary report No. 751, submitted to WHO by Bayer AG, Germany).

BOWMAN, P.B. & DAME, P.W. (1974) Gas-liquid chromatography of trichlorfon in soluble powder formulations. *J. Assoc. Off. Anal. Chem.*, **57**: 1128-1131.

BRAUN, R., SCHÖNEICH, J., WEISSFLOG, L., & DEDEK, W. (1982) Activity of organophosphorus insecticides in bacterial tests for mutagenicity and DNA repair - direct alkylation vs. metabolic activation and breakdown. 1. Butonate, vinylbutonate, trichlorfon, dichlorvos, demethyl dichlorvos and demethyl vinylbutonate. *Chem.-biol. Interact.*, **39**: 339-350.

BRODEUR, J. & DUBOIS, K.P. (1963) Comparison of acute toxicity of anticholinesterase insecticides to weanling and adult male rats. *Proc. Soc. Exp. Biol. Med.*, **114**: 509-511.

BRZHESKII, V.V. (1973) [Possibility of induction of mutations in *Drosophila melanogaster* with chlorophos.] *Med. Parazitol. Parazit. Bolezn.*, **42**: 703-706 (in Russian).

BUCHET, J.P. & LAUWERYS, R. (1970) Inhibition of rat heart diolein hydrolase and brain acetylcholinesterase by organophosphate esters *in vitro*. *Biochim. biophys. Acta.*, **218**: 369-371.

BULL, D.L. & RIDGWAY, R.L. (1969) Metabolism of trichlorfon in animals and plants. *J. agric. food Chem.*, **17**(4): 837-841.

BULSIEWICZ, H., ROZEWICKA, L., JANUSZEWSKA, H., & BAJKO, J. (1976) Aberrations of meiotic chromosomes induced in mice with insecticides. *Folia morphol. (Warsaw)*, **35**: 361-368.

CAIN, J.R. & CAIN, R.K. (1984) Effects of five insecticides on zygospore germination and growth of the green alga *Chlamydomonas moewusii*. *Bull. environ. Contam. Toxicol.*, **33**(5): 571-574.

CARERE, A., ORTALI, V.A., CARDAMONE, G., & MORPURGO, G. (1978a) Mutagenicity of dichlorvos and other structurally related pesticides in *Salmonella* and *Streptomyces*. *Chem.-biol. Interact.*, **22**: 297-308.

CARERE, A., ORTALI, V.A., CARDAMONE, G., TORRACA, A.M., & RASCHETTI, R. (1978b) Microbiological mutagenicity studies of pesticides *in vitro*. *Mutat. Res.*, **57**: 277-286.

CAROLDI, S. & LOTTI, M. (1981) Delayed neurotoxicity caused by a single massive dose of dichlorvos to adult hens. *Toxicol. Lett.*, **9**: 157-159.

CERNA, V. (1963) [Colorimetric determination of dipterex residues in foods.] *Nahrung*, **7**: 60-66 (in German).

CHAN, P.C. & PETERS, A.C. (1989) Thirteen-week subchronic dosed feed study of trichlorfon in Fischer rats and B6C3F1 mice. *Proc. Am. Assoc. Cancer Res.*, **30**: 137.

CHAPMAN, R.A. & COLE, C.M. (1982) Observations on the influence of water and soil pH on the persistence of insecticides. *J. environ. Sci. Health*, **B17**: 487-504.

CHEN, H.H., HSUEH, J.L., SIRIANNI, S.R., & HUANG, C.C. (1981) Induction of sister chromatid exchanges and cell cycle delay in cultured mammalian cells treated with eight organophosphorus pesticides. *Mutat. Res.*, **88**: 307-316.

CHEN, H.H., SIRIANNI, S.R., & HUANG, C.C. (1982) Sister chromatid exchanges in Chinese hamster cells treated with seventeen organophosphorus compounds in the presence of a metabolic system. *Environ. Mutagen.*, **4**: 621-624.

CLEMENS, G.R. & HARTNAGEL, R.E. (1986) *Critique: Assessment of the teratogenic potential of trichlorfon in mice and rats*, Elkhart, USA, Miles Laboratories, Toxicology Department, (Proprietary report submitted to WHO by Bayer AG, Germany).

CLEMENS, G.R., TROUP, C.M., & HARTNAGEL, R.E. (1990) *Teratology study in the rabbit with Dylox technical (Trichlorfon)*, Elkhart, USA, Miles Laboratories, Toxicology Department, (Proprietary report No. MTD 0134, submitted to WHO by Bayer AG, Germany).

CONRAD, R., DEDEK, W., & ENGEWALD, W. (1987) [Determination of trichlorfon in biological media and technical products following derivatization with acetic anhydride by gas chromatography]. *Fresenius Z. anal. Chem.*, **326**: 241-246 (in German).

COURTNEY, K.D. & ANDREWS, J.E. (1980) Extra ribs indicate fetotoxicity and maldevelopment. *Teratology*, **21**(2): 35A (Meeting abstract).

COURTNEY, K.D., ANDREWS, J.E., & SPRINGER, J. (1986) Assessment of teratogenic potential of trichlorfon in mice and rats. *J. environ. Sci. Health*, **B 21**: 207-227.

COX, C.L., TIMMONS, L.L., & RIDLEN, R.L. (1989) Capillary gas chromatographic analysis of trichlorfon in dosed feed formulations. *J. anal. Toxicol.*, **13**: 84-88.

CSIK, V., MOTIKA, D., & MAROSI, G.Y. (1986) Delayed neuropathy after trichlorfon intoxication. *J. Neurol. Neurosurg. Psychiatry*, **49**(2): 222.

DALDRUP, T., SUSANTO, F., & MICHALKE, P. (1981) [Combination of TLC, GLC (OV 1 and OV 17) and HPLC (RP 18) for a rapid detection of drugs, intoxicants and related compounds.] *Fresenius Z. anal. Chem.*, **308**: 413-427 (in German).

DALDRUP, T., MICHALKE, P., & BOEHME, W. (1982) A screening test for pharmaceuticals, drug and insecticides with reversed-phase liquid chromatography-retention data of 560 compounds. *Chromatogr. Newsl.*, **10**: 1-7.

DAVIS, A. (1986) Recent advances in schistomiasis. *Q. J. Med.*, **226**: 95-110.

DEDEK, W. (1968) [Degradation and residues of butonate-32p in fruits.] *Z. Naturforsch.*, **B 23**: 504-506 (in German).

DEDEK, W. (1981) Guanine N^7-alkylation in mice *in vivo* by metrifonate-discussion of possible genotoxic risk in mammals. *Acta pharmacol. toxicol.*, **Suppl.49**: 40-50.

DEDEK, W. & LOHS, K. (1970) [Alkylating effect of trichlorphon in warm blooded animals. II. Distribution of ^{14}C in organs and liver proteins of rats after application of trichlorfon-^{14}C.] *Z. Naturforsch.*, **B 25**: 1110-1113 (in German).

DEDEK, W. & SCHWARZ, H. (1966) [Metabolism and application of trichlorfon in veterinary praxis.] *Atompraxis,* **12**: 603-606 (in German).

DEDEK, W. & SCHWARZ, H. (1967) [Studies on percutaneous resorption of ^{32}P-labeled systemic organic phosphorus compounds of relatively small toxicity in cattle.] *Z. Naturforsch.*, **B 22**: 702-706 (in German).

DEDEK, W. & SCHWARZ, H. (1970a) [Residues in farm animals following the application of ^{32}P-labelled organophosphorus insecticides.] *Arch. exp. Veterinaermed*, **24**: 719-726 (in German).

DEDEK, W. & SCHWARZ, H. (1970b) [Studies of the percutaneous resorption of ^{32}P-trichlorfon and ^{32}P-dimethoate in sheep.] *Z. Naturforsch.*, **B 25**: 1193-1194 (in German).

DEDEK, W., KOCH, H., UHLENHUT, G., & BROSE, F. (1969) [Decomposition of ^{3}H-trichlorfon to dimethyl dichlorovinyl phosphate.] *Z. Naturforsch.*, **B 24**: 663-664 (in German).

DEDEK, W., LOHS, K., & GIBEL,W. (1975a) Studies on the alkylating properties of trichlorphone and dimethoate in mammals. *Environ. Qual. Saf.*, **3**(Suppl.): 648-651.

DEDEK, W., SCHEUFLER, H., & FISCHER, G.W. (1975b) Mutagenicity of desmethyltrichlorfon in the dominant lethal test in mice. *Arch. Toxicol.*, **33**: 163-168.

DEDEK, W., LOHS, K., FISCHER, G.W., & SCHMIDT, R. (1976) Alkylation of guanine in mice *in vivo* by organophosphorus insecticides. I. Trichlorfon and butonate. *Pestic. Biochem. Physiol.*, **6**: 101-110.

DEDEK, W., GEORGI, W., & GRAHL, R. (1979) Comparative degradation and metabolism of ^{32}P labeled butonate, trichlorfon and dichlorvos in crop plants. *Biochem. Physiol. Pflanzen*, **174**: 707-722.

DEDEK, W., GRAHL, R., & SCHMIDT, R. (1984) A comparative study of guanine N7-alkylation in mice *in vivo* by the organophosphorus insecticides trichlorfon, dimethoate, phosmet and bromophos. *Acta pharmacol. toxicol.*, **55**: 104-109.

DEDEK, W., WENZEL, K.D., LUFT, F., OBERLÄNDER, H., & MOTHES, B. (1987) Preconcentration of hydrophilic pesticides from aqueous solutions and extraction of residues using the polymeric sorbent Wofatil Y77. I. Preconcentration of hydrophilic pesticides from water. *Fresenius Z. anal. Chem.*, **328**: 484-486.

DEGRAEVE, N., GILOT-DELHALLE, J., COLIZZI, A., CHOLLET, M.C., MOUTSCHEN, J., & MOUTSCHEN-DAHMEN, M. (1981) Evaluation des risques génétiques d'un insecticide organophosphoré: le trichlorfon (*O,O*-diméthyl-(2,2,2 trichloro-1-hydroxy)-éthylphosphonate). *Bull. Soc. R. Sci. Liege,* **50**(1-2): 85-98.

DEGRAEVE, N., CHOLLET, M.C., & MOUTSCHEN, J. (1984a) Cytogenetic and genetic effects of subchronic treatments with organophosphorus insecticides. *Arch. Toxicol.*, **56**: 66-67.

DEGRAEVE, N., CHOLLET, M.C., & MOUTSCHEN, J. (1984b) Cytogenetic effects induced by organophosphorus pesticides in mouse spermatocytes. *Toxicol. Lett.*, **21**: 315-319.

DEGRAEVE, N., CHOLLET, M.C., & MOUTSCHEN, J. (1985) Mutagenic efficiency of organophosphorus insecticides used in combined treatments. *Environ. Health Perspect.*, **60**: 395-398.

DEGTYAREVA, L.A., POLITOVA, K.S., FOMICHENKO, E.L., & KOCHKINA, N.P. (1977) [Hygienic evaluation of the air in buildings where chlorophos-containing insecticides are processed.] *Probl. Dezinfekts Steril., Mater. Simp.*, **3**: 26-27 (in Russian).

DEICHMANN, W.B. & LAMPE, K. (1955) Dipterex, its pharmacological action. *Bull. Univ. Miami Sch. Med.*, **9**: 7-12.

DE KERGOMMEAUX, D.J., GRANT, W.F., & SANDHU, S.S. (1983) Clastogenic and physiological response of chromosomes to nine pesticides in the *Vicia faba in vivo* root tip assay system. *Mutat. Res.*, **124**: 69-84.

DÉSI, I. (1983) Neurotoxicological investigations of pesticides in animal experiments. *Neurobehav. Toxicol. Teratol.,* **5**: 503-515.

DEVINE, J.M. (1973) Determination of trichlorfon (*O,O*-Dimethyl- (2,2,2-trichloro-1-hydroxyethyl)phosphonate) in forest environmental samples. *J. agric. food Chem.*, **21**: 1095-1098.

DIVE, D., LECLERC, H., & PERSOONE, G. (1980) Pesticide toxicity on the ciliate protozoan. *Colpidium campylum*: possible consequences of the effect of pesticides in the aquatic environment. *Ecotoxicol. environ. Saf.*, **4**: 129-133.

DMITRIYEV, A.I. (1970) [Trichlorfon action on the quality of chicken slaughter products.] *Veterinariya,* **46**: 104-106 (in Russian).

DOBSON, K.J. (1977) Trichlorfon toxicity in pigs. *Aust. vet. J.*, **53**: 115-117.

DOULL, J. & DUBOIS, K.P. (1956) The effects of diets containing Dipterex on rats, (Unpublished report by Department of Pharmacology, University of Chicago).

DOULL, J., ROOT, M., VESSELINOVITCH, D., MESKAUSKAS, J., & FITCH, F. (1962a) *Chronic oral toxicity of Dylox to male and female dogs*, (Unpublished report submitted to WHO by Farbenfabriken Bayer A.G., Germany).

DOULL, J., VESSELINOVITCH, D., ROOT, M., COWAN, J., MESKAUSKAS, J., & FITCH, F. (1962b) *Chronic oral toxicity of Dylox to male and female rats*, University of Chicago, Department of Pharmacology, (Unpublished report).

DOULL, J., VESSELINOVITCH, D., ROOT, M., COWAN, J., MESKAUSKAS, J., & COWAN, J. (1965) *Chronic oral toxicity of Dylox to male and female rats*, University of Chicago, Department of Pharmacology, (Unpublished report).

DRUDGE, J.H., LYONS, E.T., & TAYLOR, E.L. (1976) Critical tests and safety studies on trichlorfon as an antiparasitic agent in the horse. *Am. J. vet. Res.*, **37**: 139-144.

DUBOIS, K.P. & COTTER, G.J. (1955) Studies on the toxicity and mechanism of action of dipterex. *Am. Med. Assoc. Arch. ind. Health,* **11**: 53-60.

DUNACHIE, J.F. & FLETCHER, W.W. (1969) An investigation of the toxicity of insecticides to birds' eggs using the egg-injection technique. *Ann. appl. Biol.*, **64**: 409-423.

DZWONKOWSKA, A. & HUBNER, H. (1986) Induction of chromosomal aberrations in the Syrian hamster by insecticides tested *in vivo*. *Arch. Toxicol.*, **58**: 152-156.

ECOBICHON, D.J. (1979) The chemical stability of trichlorfon in fresh and salt water as measured by changes in anticholinesterase potency. *Toxicol. Lett.*, **3**: 117-120.

ECOBICHON, D.J., OZERE, R.L., REID, E., & CROCKER, J.F.S. (1977) Acute fenitrothion poisoning. *Can. Med. Assoc. J.*, **116**: 377-379.

EDSON, E.F. & NOAKES, D.N. (1960) The comparative toxicity of six organophosphorus insecticides. *Toxicol. appl. Pharmacol.*, **2**: 523-539.

EL-HISSY, F.T. & ABDEL-KADER, M.I.A. (1980) Effect of five pesticides on the mycelial growth of some soil and pathogenic fungi. *Z. allg. Mikrobiol.*, **20**: 257-263.

EPSTEIN, S.S., ARNOLD, E., ANDREA, J., BASS, W., & BISHOP, Y. (1972) Detection of chemical mutagens by the dominant lethal assay in the mouse. *Toxicol. appl. Pharmacol.*, **23**: 288-325.

FAO (1982) *Second Government Consultation on International Harmonization of Pesticide Registration Requirements, Rome, 11-15 October, 1982*, Rome, Food and Agriculture Organization of the United Nations.

FAO/WHO (1972) Trichlorfon. In: *1971 Evaluations of some pesticide residues in food,* Geneva, World Health Organization, pp. 183-230 (WHO Pesticide Residues Series, No. 1).

FAO/WHO (1976) Trichlorfon. In: *1975 Evaluations of some pesticide residues in food,* Geneva, World Health Organization, pp. 379-392 (WHO Pesticide Residues Series, No. 5).

FAO/WHO (1979) Trichlorfon. In: *Pesticide residues in food: 1978 Evaluations,* Rome, Food and Agriculture Organization of the United Nations. pp. 235-255 (FAO Plant Production and Protection Paper 15 Sup.).

FAO/WHO (1986) *Codex maximum limits for pesticide residues,* Rome, Codex Alimentarius Commission, Food and Agriculture Organization of the United Nations. (CAC/Vol. XIII-Ed. 2).

FAO/WHO (1989) *Guide to Codex recommendations concerning pesticide residues. Part 8. Recommendations for methods of analysis of pesticide residues,* 4th ed., Rome, Codex Committee on Pesticide Residues, Food and Agriculture Organization of the United Nations (CAC/PR8-1989).

FECHNER, G., FUEHRER, G., & ACKERMANN, H. (1968) [Studies of milk contamination following trichlorfon treatment of milk cows.] *Monatsh. Veterinärmed.*, **23**: 529-531 (in German).

FECHNER, G., KRETZSCHMANN, F., ACKERMANN, H., & TOPFER, H. (1971) [Improved method of thin-layer chromatographic and enzymic determination of trichlorfon and dichlorvos residues in milk.] *Monatsh. Veterinärmed.*, **26**: 860-863 (in German).

FEDORENKO, A.P., ALEEVA, L.V., & TITOK, V.A. (1981) [Organophosphorus pesticide accumulation in warm-blood animals after chemical treatment of the forest.] *Vestn. Zool.*, **4**: 89-92 (in Russian).

FERREIRA, J.R. & FERNANDES, A.M.S.S. (1980) Gas-liquid chromatographic determination of organophosphorus insecticide residues in fruits and vegetables. *J. Assoc. Off. Anal. Chem.*, **63**: 517-522.

FILATOV, G.V., SIVOKHIN, P.A., & METELITSA, V.K. (1972) Trichlorfon excretion in milk. *Veterinariya,* **5**: 102 (in Russian).

FISCHER, G.W., SCHNEIDER, P., & SCHEUFLER, H. (1977) Mutagenicity of dichloroacetaldehyde and methyl-2,2- dichloro-1,1-dihydroxyethane phosphonate, possible trichlorfon metabolites. *Chem.-biol. Interact.*, **19**: 205-213.

FOURNIER, E., SONNIER, M., & DALLY, S. (1978) Detection and assay of organophosphate pesticides in human blood by gas chromatography. *Clin. Toxicol.*, **12**: 457-462.

FRANCIS, B.M., METCALF, R.L., & HANSEN, L.G. (1985) Toxicity of organophosphorus esters to laying hens after oral and dermal administration. *J. environ. Sci. Health,* **B 20**: 74-95.

FROHLICH, D.R., BOEKER, E.A., & BRINDLEY, W.A. (1990) The kinetics and inhibition of *p*-nitrophenylacetate-hydrolising esterases in a solitary bee, *Megachile rotundata* (Fab.). Xenobiotica, **20**(5): 481-487.

GAINES, T.B. (1969) Acute toxicity of pesticides. *Toxicol. appl. Pharmacol.*, **14**: 515-534.

GARRETT, N.E., STACK, H.F., & WATERS, M.D. (1986) Evaluation of the genetic activity profiles of 65 pesticides. *Mutat. Res.*, **168**: 301-325.

GETZ, M.E. & WHEELER, H.G. (1968) Thin-layer chromatography of organophosphorus insecticides with several adsorbents and ternary solvent systems. *J. Assoc. Off. Anal. Chem.*, **51**: 1101-1107.

GIANG, P.A. & CASWELL, R.L. (1957) Polarographic determination of *O,O*-dimethyl 2,2,2-trichloro-1-hydroxyethylphosphonate(Bayer L13/59). *J. agric. food Chem.*, **5**: 753-754.

GIANG, P.A., BARTHEL, W.F., & HALL, S.A. (1954) Colorimetric determination of *O,O*-dialkyl 1-hydroxyphosphonates derived from chloral. *J. agric. food Chem.*, **2**: 1281-1284.

GIBEL, W., VON, LOHS, K.H., WILDNER, G.P., & ZIEBARTH, D. (1971) [Experimental studies on hepatotoxic and carcinogenic activity of organophosphorus compounds, Trichlorfon.] *Arch. Geschwülstforsch.*, **37**: 303-312 (in German).

GIBEL, W., VON LOHS, K.H., WILDNER, G.P., ZIEBARTH, D., & STIEGLITS, R. (1973) [Experimental study on cancerogenic haematotoxic and hepatotoxic activity of organophosphorus pesticides.] *Arch. Geschwülstforsch,* **41**: 311-328 (in German).

GILOT-DELHALLE, J., COLIZZI, A., MOUTSCHEN, J., & MOUTSCHEN-DAHMEN, M. (1983) Mutagenicity of some organophosphorus compounds at the ADE6 locus of *Schizosaccharomyces pombe. Mutat. Res.*, **117**: (1-2) 139-148.

GINGERICH, D.A. & MIA, A.S. (1981) Clinical toxicosis and erythrocyte cholinesterase inhibition of trichlorfon combined with mebendazole in horses. *Am. J. vet. Res.*, **42**: 1645-1650.

GIOVANOLI-JAKUBCZAK, T., FITAK, B., & CHODKOWSKI, J. (1971) Photolysis of Dipterex and DDVP under the influence of UV irradiation. *Rocz. Chem.*, **45(4)**: 689-694.

GLUCKMAN, J.C., BARCELO, D., DE JONG, G.J., FREI, R.W., MARIS, F.A., & BRINKMAN, U.A.T. (1986) Improved design and applications of an on-line thermionic detector for narrow-bore liquid chromatography. *J. Chromatogr.*, **367**: 35-44.

GONCHARUK, E.I., PERELYGIN, V.M., & MELENEVSKAYA, A.V. (1978) [Analysis of migration of the chemicals from the soil into the atmosphere.] *Gig. i Sanit.*, **43**: 41-45 (in Russian).

GRAHL, K., HORN, H., & HALLEBACH, R. (1981) [Effect of butonate, trichlorfon and dichlorvos on plankton populations.] *Acta hydrochim. hydrobiol.*, **9**: 147-161 (in German).

GRIFFIN, T.B. (1988) *Safety evaluation and tumorigenesis of trichlorfon in Rhesus monkeys: A ten-year study*. Alamogordo, New Mexico, White Sands Research Center, (Proprietary study report No. 800108 submitted to WHO by Bayer AG, Germany).

GROMYSZ-KALKOWSKA, K., SZUBARTOWSKA, E., & KACZANOWSKA, E. (1985) Peripheral blood in the Japanese quail (*Coturnix coturnix japonica*) in acute poisoning by different insecticides. *Comp. Biochem. Physiol.*, **C81**: 290-312.

GROMYSZ-KALKOWSKA, K., SZUBARTOWSKA, E., SULIKOWSKA, J., & TROCEWICZ, K. (1985) Peripheral blood changes of the Japanese quail (*Coturnix coturnix japonica*) following repeated small doses of trichlorfon. *Bull. environ. Contam. Toxicol.*, **35**: 757-766.

GRUNDMANN, E. & HOBIK, H.P. (1966) *Bay 15922/2 year feeding experiment in rats/histology* (Unpublished report submitted to WHO by Farbenfabriken Bayer AG, Germany).

GRYGIEREK, E. & WASILEWSKA, B.E. (1981) The effect of Foschlor (organic phosphorous acid esters) on zooplankton and benthos of fish ponds. *Ekol. Pol.*, **29**: 257-270.

GUTH, J.A. (1967) [Thin-layer chromatographic separation scheme for insecticidally active phosphoric acid esters.] *Pflanzenschutzberichte,* **35**: 129-143 (in German).

HAGAN, E.C., JENNER, P.M., & JONES, W.I. (1971) Increased lethal effects of acutely administered anticholinesterases in female rats prefed with similar agents. *Toxicol. appl. Pharmacol.*, **18**: 235-237.

HALEY, T.J., HARMER, J.H., HARMON, J.R., & DOOLEY, K.L. (1975) Estimation of the LD_1 and extrapolation of the $LD_{0.1}$ for five organophosphate pesticides. *Arch. Toxicol.*, **34**: 103-109.

HALLAK, M. & GIACOBINI, E. (1987) A comparison of the effects of two inhibitors on brain cholinesterase. *Neuropharmacology,* **26**: 521-530.

HALLAK, M. & GIACOBINI, E. (1989) Physostigmine, tacrine, and metrifonate: The effect of multiple doses on acetylcholine metabolism in rat brain. *Neuropharmacology*, **28**: 199-206.

HAMEED, S.F., SURI, S.M., & KASHYAP, N.P. (1980) Toxicity and persistence of residues of some organophosphorus insecticides applied for the control of *Dacus cucurbitae Coquillet* on the fruits of cucumber. *Indian J. agric. Sci.*, **50**: 73-77.

HANNA, P.J. & DYER, K.F. (1975) Mutagenicity of organophosphorus compounds in bacteria and *Drosophila. Mutat. Res.*, **28**: 405-420.

HANNA, S., BASMY, K., OSAIMA, S., SHOEB, S.M., & AWNY, A.Y. (1966) Effects of administration of an organophosphorus compound as an antibilharzial agent with special reference to plasma cholinesterase. *Br. med. J.*, **1**: 1390-1392.

HANSEN, H.J., KRONEVI, T., & BJÖRKLUND, N.E. (1978) On cerebellar hypoplasia in domestic animals. In: 13th Nord. Vet. Congress Abo, July 1978.

HASHIMOTO, Y., OKUBO, E., ITO, T., YAMAGUCHI, M., & TANAKA, S. (1982) Changes in susceptibility of carp to several pesticides with growth. *J. pestic. Sci.*, **7**: 457-461.

HASSAN, A. & ZAYED, S.M.A.D. (1965) Metabolism of organophosphorus insecticides. III. Fate of the methyl groups of Dipterex *in vivo. Can. J. Biochem.*, **43**: 1271-1275.

HASSAN, A., ZAYED, S.M.A.D., & HASHISH, S. (1965) Metabolism of organophosphorus insecticides. VI. Mechanism of detoxification of Dipterex in the rat. *Biochem. Pharmacol.*, **14**: 1692-1694.

HATTORI, K. (1974) [Toxicological studies on the effect of chemicals on birds (part 2). Oral acute toxicity of three organophosphate insecticides in the common pigeon.] *Hokkaidoritsu Eisei Kenkyusho Ho,* **24**: 154 (in Japanese).

HAYES, R.H. (1988) *Oncogenicity study of technical grade trichlorfon with mice,* Stillwell, Kansas, Mobay Corporation (Proprietary study report No. 1039 submitted to WHO by Bayer AG, Germany).

HAYES, R.H. (1989) *Chronic toxicity/Oncogenicity study of technical grade trichlorfon (Dylox®) with rats,* Stillwell, Kansas, Mobay Corporation (Proprietary study report No. 1108, submitted to WHO by Bayer AG, Germany).

HAYES, W.J. Jr (1982) *Pesticides studied in man,* Baltimore, Maryland, Williams & Wilkins Co., pp. 351-356.

HAYES, W.J. Jr & LAWS, E.R. Jr (1991) Fenitrothion. In: Handbook of pesticide toxicology, New York Academic Press, pp. 1020-1023.

HERBOLD, B. (1979a) *Micronucleus test on mouse to evaluate L 13/59 (Trichlorfon) for potential mutagenic effects,* Wuppertal-Elberfeld, Bayer AG, Institute of Toxicology, (Proprietary report No. 8505, submitted to WHO by Bayer AG, Germany).

HERBOLD, B. (1979b) *L 13/59 (Trichlorfon) -Dominant lethal study on male mouse to test for mutagenic effects,* Wuppertal-Elberfeld, Bayer AG, Institute of Toxicology, (Proprietary report No. 8745, submitted to WHO by Bayer AG, Germany).

HIERONS, R. & JOHNSON, M.K. (1978) Clinical and toxicological investigations of a case of delayed neuropathy in man after acute poisoning by an organophosphorus pesticide. *Arch. Toxicol.*, **40**: 279-284.

HINTON, M.J. & EVERSOLE, A.G. (1980) Toxicity and tolerance studies with yellow-phase eels: five chemicals. *Prog. Fish Cult.*, **42**: 201-203.

HIRAMATSU, R. & FURUTANI, F. (1977) [Persistence of sprayed insecticides in head vegetables.] *Bull. Yamaguchi-ken agric. Explor. Stn*, **28**: 159-163 (in Japanese).

HIRAMATSU, R. & FURUTANI, F. (1978) [Persistence of sprayed malathion and trichlorfon in grape berries and grape products.] *Bull. Yamaguchi-ken agric. Explor. Stn,* **30**: 37-44 (in Japanese).

HOFER, W. (1981) Chemistry of metrifonate and dichlorvos. *Acta pharmacol. Scand.*, **49**(Suppl.5): 7-14.

HOFFMANN, K., RUF, J., & MAGER, H. (1988) *Study of the chronic toxicity to Rhesus monkeys, oral administration for 26 weeks (oral intubation tube administration).* Wuppertal, Bayer AG, (Proprietary study report No. 90237, submitted to WHO by Bayer, AG, Germany).

HOLMSTEDT, B., NORDGREN, I., SANDOZ, M., & SUNDWALL, A. (1978) Metrifonate, summary of toxicological and pharmacological information available. *Arch. Toxicol.*, **41**: 3-29.

HU, X., LU, Y., XUE, S., LING, Y., & GU, X. (1986) Toxicity of dipterex: A field study. *Br. J. ind. Med.*, **43**: 414-419.

IARC (1983) Trichlorfon. In: *Miscellaneous pesticides*, Lyon, International Agency for Research on Cancer, pp. 207-231 (IARC Monographs on the evaluation of the carcinogenic risk of chemicals to humans, Vol. 30).

IARC (1987) *Overall evaluations of carcinogenicity: An updating of IARC Monographs volumes 1 to 42*, Lyon, International Agency for Research on Cancer, p. 73 (IARC Monographs on the evaluation of the carcinogenic risk of chemicals to humans, Suppl. 7).

IARC (in press) *Re-evaluation of dichlorvos*. Lyon, France, IARC (IARC Monographs on the evaluation of the carcinogenic risk of chemicals to humans).

IMANAKA, M., MATSUNAGA, K., & ISHIDA, T. (1981) [Gas-liquid chromatographic determination of trichlorfon (Dipterex) in livestock products using a flame photometric detector.] *J. Food Hyg. Soc. Jpn.*, **22**: 472-478 (in Japanese).

IRPTC/GKNT (1983) In: Izmerov, N.F., ed. *Trichlorfon,* Moscow, Centre of International Projects, GKNT, 24 pp. (Scientific Reviews of Soviet Literatures on Toxicity and Hazards of Chemicals No. 33).

ISAAC, I.G., SHAFIC, M.T., TANTAWY, G., & EL-KHISHEN, S.A. (1965) Trichlorfon residues on cotton. *Alexandria J. agric. Res.*, **14**: 3-4.

ISHIDATE, M., Jr, SOFUNI, T., & YOSHIKAWA, K. (1981) Chromosomal aberration tests *in vitro* as a primary screening tool for environmental mutagens and/or carcinogens. *Gann*, **27**: 95-108.

ISHIZAKA, T., SEKITA, H., SUZUKI, T., & SAITOU, Y. (1986) Analytical method for trichlorfon in agricultural foods by gas chromatography. *Shokuhin Eiseigaku Zasshi,* **27**: 288-295.

IVANOVA, L.N. & MOLOZHANOVA, E.G. (1974) [Kinetics of the transformation of some pesticides in the soil.] *Khim. Sel'sk. Khoz.*, **12**: 363-365 (in Russian).

IWATA, Y., DUSH, M.E., CARMAN, G.E., & GUNTHER, F.A. (1979) Worker environment research, residues from carbaryl, chlorobenzilate, dimethoate and trichlorfon applied to citrus trees. *J. agric. food Chem.*, **27**: 1141-1145.

JAPAN PLANT PROTECTION ASSOCIATION (1985) [Pesticides handbook], Tokyo, Japan Plant Protection Association (in Japanese).

JAPAN PLANT PROTECTION ASSOCIATION (1986) [Production statistics of major pesticides - fenitrothion and trichlorfon.] In: [Pesticides handbook], Tokyo, Japan Plant Protection Association, p. 54 (in Japanese).

JAPAN PLANT PROTECTION ASSOCIATION (1988) [Production statistics of major pesticides - fenitrothion and trichlorfon.] In: [Pesticides handbook], Tokyo, Japan Plant Protection Association, p. 57 (in Japanese).

JAPAN PLANT PROTECTION ASSOCIATION (1989) [Production statistics of major pesticides - fenitrothion and trichlorfon.] In: [Pesticides handbook], Tokyo, Japan Plant Protection Association, p. 60 (in Japanese).

JOHANSEN, C.A. (1972) Toxicity of field-weathered insecticide residues to four kinds of bees. *Environ. Entomol.*, **1**: 393-394.

JOHNSON, M.K. (1981) Delayed neurotoxicity - do trichlorfon and/or dichlorvos cause delayed neuropathy in man or in test animals? *Acta pharmacol. toxicol.*, **49**(Suppl.V): 87-98.

JOHNSON, M.K. (1990) Organophosphates and delayed neuropathy - is NTE alive and well? *Toxicol. appl. Pharmacol.*, **102**: 385-399.

JONES, D.C.L., SIMMON, V.F., MORTELMANS, K.E., MITCHELL, A.D., EVANS, E.L., JOTZ, M.M., RICCIO, E.S., ROBINSON, D.E., & KIRKHART, B.A. (1982) In vitro *mutagenicity studies of environmental chemicals*, Washington, DC, National Technical Information Service.

KAWACHI, T., KOMATSU, T., KADA, T., ISHIDATE, M., Jr, SASAKI, M., SUGIYAMA, T., & TAZIMA, Y. (1980) Results of recent studies on the relevance of various short-term screening tests in Japan. In: *The predictive value of short-term screening tests in carcinogenicity evaluation*, Amsterdam, Elsevier/North-Holland Biomedical Press, pp. 253-267.

KAWAI, M., YOSHIDA, M., IYATOMI, A., KOYAMA, M., & KANEKO, Y. (1982) [Exposure of spray-operators to trichlorfon.] *Nippon koshu Eisei Zasshi*, **29**: 165-171 (in Japanese).

KAWAMOTO, K. & URANO, K. (1989) Parameters for predicting fate of organochlorine pesticides in the environment (I) Octanol-water and air-water partition coefficients. *Chemosphere*, **18**: 1987-1996.

KIMMERLE, G. & LOSER, E. (1974) Delayed neurotoxicity of organophosphorus compounds and copper concentration in the serum of hens. *Environ. Qual. Saf.*, **3**: 173-178.

KIMMERLE, G. (1975a) *Acute inhalation toxicity study on rats* (Unpublished report No. 5581 from Bayer AG, Germany).

KIMMERLE, G. (1975b) *Subacute inhalation toxicity study on rats* (Unpublished report No. 5582 from Bayer AG, Germany).

KIMURA, S., YOKOTE, M., & MATIDA, Y. (1971) Study on the toxicity of agricultural control chemicals in relation to freshwater fisheries management No.6 Chronic toxicity of dieldrin, lindane and dipterex to cherry salmon fingerlings. *Bull. Freshwater Fish. Res. Lab.*, **21**: 107-116.

KIRALY, J., SZENTESI, I., RUZICSKA, M., & CZEIZE, A. (1979) Chromosome studies in workers producing organophosphate insecticides. *Arch. environ. Contam. Toxicol.*, **8**: 309-319.

KLISENKO, M.A. & PISMENNAYA, M.V. (1979) [Photochemical conversion of organophosphorus pesticides in the air.] *Gig. Tr. prof. Zabol.*, 56-58 (in Russian).

KNOX, B., ASKAA, J., BASSE, A., BITSCH, V., ESKILDSEN, M., MANDRUP, M., OTTOSEN, H.E., OVERBY, E., PEDERSEN, K.B., & RASMUSSEN, F. (1978) Congenital ataxia and tremor with cerebellar hypoplasia in piglets borne by sows treated with Neguvon® vet (Metrifonate, Trichlorfon) during pregnancy. *Nord. vet. Med.*, **30**: 538-545.

KOKOSZKA, L.C. & FLOOD, J.W. (1989) Environmental management handbook. Appendix 15: Common chemical toxicants found at hazardous waste sites, New York, Basel, Marcel Dekker.

KONRAD, H., GABRIO, T., & PENNER, G. (1975) [Pesticide contamination of milk and milk products.] *Milchforsch-Milchprax.* **17**: 67-69 (in German).

KOWALSKI, R.L., CLEMENS, G.R., BARE, J.J., & HARTNAGEL, R.E. Jr, (1987) *A teratology study with Dylox®, technical (Trichlorfon) in the rat.* Elkhart, USA, Miles Laboratories, Toxicology Department, (Proprietary report No. MTD0017, submitted to WHO by Bayer AG, Germany).

KRONEVI, T., HANSEN, H.J., & JONSSON, O.J. (1975) Cerebellar hypoplasia of unknown etiology in pigs. *Vet. Rec.*, **May 1975**: 403- 404.

KRUSTEV, E., KONSTANTINOV, P., & VASILEV, V. (1976) [The effect of subtoxic doses of dipterex on guinea pigs.] *Vet.-Med. Nauki,* **13**(1): 48-51 (in Russian).

KURINNIY, A.I. (1975) [Comparative investigation of the cytogenetic effect of certain organophosphorus pesticides.] *Genetika,* **11**: 64-69 (in Russian).

KURINNIY, A.I. & PILINSKAYA, M.A. (1977) [Cytogenetic acticity of the pesticides imidan, dipterex and gardona in cultured human lymphocytes.] *Genetika*, **13**: 337-339 (in Russian).

KURTZ, D.A. & STUDHOLME, C.R. (1974) Recovery of trichlorfon (Dylox®) and carbaryl (Sevin®) in songbirds following spraying of forest for gypsy moth. *Bull. environ. Contam. Toxicol.*, **11**: 78-84.

KUZMENKO, N.M., DIDENKO, G.G., KURINNIY, A.L., MARTSON, L.V., PETROVSKAYA, O.G., PILINSKAYA, M.A., & SHEPELSKAYA, N.R. (1980) [Long-term health effects of pesticides.] *Gig. i Sanit.*, **45**: 88-89 (in Russian).

LAMB, M.J. (1977) Mutagenicity tests with metrifonate in *Drosophilla melanogaster. Mutat. Res.*, **56**: 157-162.

LANGE, C. (1980) [Identification of a metabolite of trichlorfon.] *Z. Chem.*, **20**: 446-447 (in German).

LEBRUN, A. & CERF, C. (1960) Note préliminaire sur la toxicité pour l'homme d'un insecticide organophosphoré (Dipterex). *Bull. World Health Organ.*, **22**: 579-582.

LEHOTZKY, K. (1982) Effect of pesticides on central and peripheral nervous system function in rats. *Neurobehav. Toxicol. Teratol.*, **4**: 665-669.

LIVINGSTON, R.J. (1977) Review of current literature concerning the acute and chronic effects of pesticides on aquatic organisms. *CRC Crit. Rev. environ. Control,* **November 1977**: 325-351.

LOGVINENKO, V.F. & MORGUN, V.V. (1978) Study of mutagenic action of certain pesticides on spring durum wheat. *Cytol. Genet. (USSR)*, **12**: 207-212.

LORENZ, W., HENGLEIN, A., & SCHRADER, G. (1955) The new insecticide *O,O*-dimethyl 2,2,2-trichloro-1-hydroxy ethylphosphonate. *J. Am. Chem. Soc.*, **77**: 2554-2556.

LORKE, D. & LOSER, E. (1966) *Chronic toxicological studies on rats* (Unpublished report submitted to WHO by Farbenfabriken Bayer AG, Germany).

LOSER, E. (1969) [Propagation trials in rats.] (Unpublished report submitted to WHO by Farbenfabriken Bayer AG, Germany) (in German).

LOSER, E. (1970) *Bay 15992/Chronic toxicological studies on dogs* (Unpublished report submitted by Farbenfabriken Bayer AG, Germany).

LU, Y.P., LU, P., XUE, S., & GU, X. (1984) Investigation on the chronic effects of dipterex in occupational exposure. *Med. Lav.*, **75**: 376-384.

MCCANN, J.A. & JASPER, R.L. (1972) Vertebral damage to bluegills exposed to acutely toxic levels of pesticides. *Trans. Amer. Fish. Soc.*, **101**: 317-322.

MCGREGOR, D.B., BROWN, A., CATTANACH, P., EDWARDS, I., MCBRIDE, D., RIACH, C., & CASPARY, W.J. (1988) Responses of the L5178Y tk+/tk- mouse lymphoma cell forward mutation assay: III. 72 coded chemicals. *Environ. mol. Mutagen.*, **12**(1): 85-154.

MACDOUGALL, D. (1964) Dylox. In: Zweig, G. ed. *Analytical methods for pesticides and plant growth regulators*, New York, London, Academic Press, Vol. 2, pp. 199-208.

MACHEMER, L. (1979a) *Trichlorfon - Evaluation for embryotoxic and teratogenic effects on orally dosed rats,* Wuppertal-Elberfeld, Bayer AG, Institute of Toxicology (Proprietary report No. 8400, submitted to WHO by Bayer AG, Germany).

MACHEMER, L. (1979b) *Trichlorfon - Evaluation for embryotoxic and teratogenic effects on orally dosed rabbits*, Wuppertal-Elberfeld, Bayer AG, Institute of Toxicology (Proprietary report No. 8430, submitted to WHO by Bayer AG, Germany).

MACHEMER, L. (1981) Chronic toxicity of metrifonate. *Acta pharmacol. toxicol.*, **49**(Suppl.V): 15-28.

MAGALHAES, M.J.A., FERREIRA, J.R., FRUTUOSA, L., & TAINHA, A.A. (1989) Study of the disappearance of endosulfan, parathion, trichlorfon, and pirimicarb from broccoli and portuguese cabbage. *Pestic. Sci.*, **27**: 23-31.

MAHENDRU, V.K. & AGARWAL, R.A. (1981) Changes in carbohydrate metabolism in various organs of the snail, *Lymnaea acuminata* following exposure to trichlorfon. *Acta pharmacol. toxicol.*, **48**: 377-381.

MANDOUL, R., DUBOS, M., DE COURNUAUD, M., & MOULINIER, CL. (1967) *In vitro* effects of organophosphorus compounds on the Portugese oyster, some molluscs, and freshwater microplankton. *Bull. Soc. Pathol. Exot.*, **60**: 568-580.

MARKING, L.L. & MAUCK, W.L. (1975) Toxicity of paired mixtures of candidate forest insecticides to rainbow trout. *Bull. environ. Contam. Toxicol.*, **13**: 518-523.

MARTSON, L.V. & VORONINA, V.M. (1976) Experimental study of the effect of a series of phosphoroorganic pesticides (dipterex and imidan) on embryogenesis. *Environ. Health Perspect.*, **13**: 121-125.

MATKOVICS, B., SZABO, L., MINDSZENTY, L., & IVAN, J. (1980) The effects of organophosphate pesticides on some liver enzymes and lipid peroxidation. *Gen. Pharmacol.*, **11**: 353-356.

MATKOVICS, B., SZABO, L., IVAN, J., & GAAL, I. (1983) Some further data on the effects of two organophosphate pesticides on the oxidative metabolism in the liver. *Gen. Pharmacol.*, **124**: 689-691.

MATTON, P. & LAHAM, Q.N. (1969) Effect of the organophosphate Dylox on rainbow trout larvae. *J. Fish. Res. Board Can.*, **26**: 2193-2200.

MELNIKOV, N.N., VORONKOVA, V.V., VORONTSOVA, N.A., GUNAR, M.I., SUPIN, G.S., MOROZOVA, T.N., SHCHERBATYKH, YU. I., & SHVETSOVA-SHILVOSKAYA, K.D. (1975) [Identification of impurities in technical chlorofos.] *Khim. Sel'sk. Khoz.*, **13**: 142-145 (in Russian).

MENDOZA, C.E. (1973) Analysis of pesticides by the thin-layer chromatographic-enzyme inhibition technique. *Residue Rev.*, **50**: 43- 72.

METCALF, R.L., FUKUTO, T.R., & MARCH, R.B. (1959) Toxic action of Dipterex and DDVP to the house fly. *J. econ. Entomol.*, **52**: 44-49.

MIHAIL, F. (1985) *L 13/59 (Trichlorfon) - Study for skin-sensitizing effect on guinea-pigs,* Wuppertal-Elberfeld, Bayer AG, Institute of Toxicology (Proprietary report No. 13323, submitted to WHO by Bayer AG, Germany).

MIHAIL, F. (1986a) *L 13/59 (Trichlorfon) - Study for skin-sensitizing effect on guinea-pigs in the open epicutaneous test*, Wuppertal-Elberfeld, Bayer AG, Institute of Toxicology (Proprietary report No. 14348, submitted to WHO by Bayer AG, Germany).

MIHAIL, F. (1986b) *L 13/59 (Trichlorfon) - Skin sensitizing effect - an evaluation,* Wuppertal-Elberfeld, Bayer AG, Institute of Toxicology, (Proprietary statement 11 March 1986, submitted to WHO by Bayer AG, Germany).

MIYAMOTO, J. (1959) Non-enzymatic conversion of Dipterex into DDVP and their inhibitory action on enzymes. *Botyu-Kagaku*, **24**: 130-137.

MIYAMOTO, J. (1961) Studies on the mode of action of Dipterex. II. New glucuronides obtained from the urine of rabbit following administration of Dipterex. *Agric. biol. Chem.*, **25**: 566-572.

MIYATA, T. & SAITO, T. (1973) [Metabolism of NS 2662 (*O,O*-dimethyl-2,2-dichloro-1-hydroxyethylphosphonate).] *Botyu-Kagaku,* **38**: 81-86 (in Japanese).

MOLLHOFF, E. (1971) Determination of trichlorfon and fenthion residues in animals of different species. *Pestic. Sci.*, **2**: 179-181.

MONSON, M.H. & ALEXANDER, K. (1984) Metrifonate in pregnancy. *Trans. R. Soc. Trop. Med. Hyg.*, **78**: 565.

MORIYA, M., OHTA, T., WATANABE, K., MIYAZAWA, T., KATA, K., & SHIRASU, Y. (1983) Further mutagenicity studies on pesticides in bacterial reversion assay systems. *Mutat. Res.*, **116**: 185-216.

MORPURGO, G., AULICINO, F., BIGNAMI, M., CONTI, L., VELCICH, A. & MONTALENTI, S.G. (1977) Relationship between structure and mutagenicity dichlorvos and other pesticides. *Lincei Rend. Sci. fis. mat. nat.*, **62**: 692-701.

MOUTSCHEN-DAHMEN, J. (1981) Metrifonate and dichlorvos cytogenetic investigations. *Acta pharmacol. toxicol.*, **49**(Suppl.): 29- 39.

MÜHLMANN, R. & SCHRADER, G. (1957) [Hydrolysis of the phosphoric acid ester insecticide.] *Z. Naturforsch.*,, **B12**: 196-208 (in German).

NAGAYAMA, T., MAKI, T., KAN, K., MAKI, M., & NISHIMA, T. (1986) Survey of pesticide residues in vegetables and fruits. *Ann. Rep. Tokyo Metrop. Res. Lab. P.H.*, **37:** 173-183 (in Japanese).

NAGAYAMA, T., MAKI, T., IIDA, M., KAN, K., & NISHIMA, T. (1987) Survey of pesticide residues in vegetables and fruits. *Ann. Rep. Tokyo Metrop. Res. Lab. P.H.*, **38:** 222-228 (in Japanese).

NAGAYAMA, T., MAKI, T., IIDA, M., KAN, K., KAWAI, Y., & NISHIMA, T. (1988) Survey of pesticide residues in vegetables and fruits. *Ann. Rep. Tokyo Metrop. Res. Lab. P.H.*, **39:** 130-138 (in Japanese).

NAGAYAMA, T., MAKI, T., IIDA, M., KAN, K., KAWAI, Y., & NISHIMA, T. (1989) Survey of pesticide residues in vegetables and fruits. *Ann. Rep. Tokyo Metrop. Res. Lab. P.H.*, **40:** 155-162 (in Japanese).

NAGY, Z.S., MILE, I., & ANTONI, F. (1975) The mutagenic effect of pesticides on *Escherichia coli WP2 try. Acta Microbiol. Acad. Sci. Hung.*, **22**: 309-314.

NAISHTEIN, S.Ya. (1976) [Trichlorfon and malathion tolerances in soil.] *Khim. Sel'sk. Khoz.*, **14**: 32-34 (in Russian).

NAISHTEIN, S.Ya., ZHULINSKAYA, V.A., & YUROVSKAYA, E.M. (1973) [Stability of certain organophosphorous pesticides in soil.] *Gig. i Sanit.*, 42-45 (in Russian).

NAKAHARA, T., TAKASE, I., KAWAGOE, I., KUBOTA, T., & SAITO, T. (1972) [Residues of trichlorfon and its metabolites in fresh milk.] *Bochu-kagaku*, **37**: 149-154 (in Japanese).

NAKAHARA, T., TAKASE, I., & YOSHIMOTO, T. (1973) [Residues of trichlorfon in eel and carp.] *Noyaku Kagaku*, **1**(2): 75-76 (in Japanese).

NAKAMURA, T. & UEDA, T. (1967) Studies on the mechanisms of the monofluoroacetanilides poisoning to mammals; Part VIII. Organophosphorous compounds as a specific inhibitor to fluoroacetanilide amidohydrolase. *Agric. biol. Chem.*, **31**: 1288-1293.

NEHEZ, M., SELYPES, A., & SCHEUFLER, H. (1982) Mutagenic effect of trichlorphon and dimethoate on mouse bone marrow cells *in vivo*. *Wiss. Z. Martin-Luther-Univ. Halle-Wittenberg*, **31**(2): 57- 62.

NEHEZ, M., HUSZTA, E., MAZZAG, E., SCHEUFLER, H., SCHNEIDER, P., & FISCHER, G.W. (1987) Cytogenetic, genetic, and embryotoxicity studies with dimethyl-2,2,2,-trichloro-1-(2,2,2-trichloro-1-hydroxy- ethoxy)-ethylphosphonate, a hypothetical impurity in technical grade trichlorfon. *Ecotoxicol. environ. Saf.*, **13**: 216-224.

NEPOKLONOV, A.A. & BUKSHTYNOV, V.I. (1971) [Trichlorfon release time from sheep after aerosol treatment.] *Tr. Vses. Nauchn. Issled. Inst. Sanit.*, **39**: 200-202 (in Russian).

NEPOKLONOV, A.A. & METELITSA, V.K. (1970) [Hypoderminchlorofos used in the prophylaxis of the *hypodermatidae*.] *Veterinariya*, **46**: 70- 72 (in Russian).

NIEDZIELLA, S.W., GÖPEL, W., & BANZHAF, E. (1985) [Acute alkylphosphate poisoning (Trichlorfon) with delayed polyneuropathy.] *Z. gesamte inn. Med.*, **40**(8): 237-239 (in German).

NIKOLAYEV, P.I. (1972) [Distribution of trichlorfon and amidophos in horses and the secretion of those compounds with mare's milk.] *Tr. Vses. Nauchn. Issled. Vet. Sanit.*, **44**: 91-98 (in Russian).

NISHIUCHI, Y. (1977) [Acute toxicity of pesticide formulations to *Cyprinus carpio* at 5 different temperatures.] *Suisan Zoshoku*, **24**: 140-145 (in Japanese).

NISHIUCHI, Y. (1979a) [Acute toxicity of pesticide formulations to *Cyprinus carpio* .] *Suisan Zoshoku*, **27**: 36-41 (in Japanese).

NISHIUCHI, Y. (1979b) [Acute toxicity of pesticide formulations to *Daphnia pulex*.] *Suisan Zoshoku*, **27**: 42-47 (in Japanese).

NISHIUCHI, Y. (1979c) [Acute toxicity of pesticide formulations to *Daphnia carinata*.] *Suisan Zoshoku*, **27**: 119-124 (in Japanese).

NISHIUCHI, Y. (1981) [Evaluation of the effect of pesticides on some aquatic organisms. I. Effect of pesticides on some aquatic insects.] *Seitai Kagaku*, **4**: 31-46 (in Japanese).

NISHIUCHI, Y. & ASANO, K. (1979) [Acute toxicity of pesticide formulations to *Cloeon dipterum*.] *Suisan Zoshoku*, **27**: 48-55 (in Japanese).

NISHIUCHI, Y. & YOSHIDA, K. (1972) Toxicity of pesticides to fresh water snails. *Bull. agric. Chem. Insp. Stn.*, **12**: 86-92.

NORDGREN, I. (1981) Quantitation of metrifonate and dichlorvos in blood and tissues by gas chromatography - mass spectrophotometry. *Fundam. appl. Toxicol.*, **1**: 230-237.

NORDGREN, I., BERGSTRÖM, M., HOLMSTEDT, B., & SANDOZ, M. (1978) Transformation and action of Metrifonate. *Arch. Toxicol.*, **41**: 31-41.

NORDGREN, I., HOLMSTEDT, B., BENGTSSON, E., & FINKEL, Y. (1980) Plasma levels of metrifonate and dichlorvos during treatment of schistosomiasis with bilarcil. *Am. J. trop. Med. Hyg.*, **29**(3): 426-430.

NORDGREN, I., BENGTSSON, E., HOLMSTEDT, B., & PETTERSSON, B.M. (1981) Levels of metrifonate and dichlorvos in plasma and erythrocytes during treatment of schistosomiasis with bilarcil. *Acta pharmacol. toxicol.*, **49**(Suppl.V): 79-86.

OLAJOS, E.J. & ROSENBLUM, I. (1981) Membrane-bound and soluble esterase activities in various hen brain regions after diisopropyl phosphorofluoridate and trichlorfon treatment. *Neurotoxicology*, **2**: 463- 470.

OLAJOS, E.J., ROSENBLUM, I., COULSTON, F., & STROMINGER, N. (1979) The dose response relationship of trichlorfon neurotoxicity in hens. *Ecotoxicol. environm. Saf.*, **3**: 245-255.

ORDOG, V. (1979) [Effect of organophosphate insecticides on green algae.] *Hydrol. Kozl.*, **59**: 36-42 (in Hungarian).

OSBORNE, B.G., BARRETT, G.M., LAAL-KHOSHAB, A., & WILLIS, K.H. (1989) The occurrence of pesticide residues in UK home-grown and imported wheat. *Pestic. Sci.*, **27**: 103-109.

OTTO, D., BEHNISCH, I., PFEIFFER, G., DEDEK, W., & GEORGI, W. (1980) Metabolismus von Trichlorfon in sensiblen und resistenten Fliegen, *Musca domestica L.*, *Arch. Phytopathol. Pflanzenschutz*, **16**: 397-411.

PAIK, S.G. & LEE, S.Y. (1977) Genetic effects of pesticides in the mammalian cells. 1. Induction of micronucleus. *Tongmul Hakhoe Chi*, **20**: 19-28.

PAKHLEVANYAN, A.S., PIRUMOV, S.S., DRAGA, O.N., ZORABYAN, S.L., & CHARCHOGLYAN, M.S. (1979) [Effect of the treatment of cow with trichlorfon on some milk composition indexes.] *Molochn. Prom-st'*, **7**: 42-44 (in Russian).

PANDA, B.B. & SHARMA, C.B.S.R. (1980) Cytogenetic hazards from agricultural chemicals. 3. Monitoring the cytogenetic activity of trichlorfon and dichlorvos in *Hordeum vulgare*. *Mutat. Res.*, **78**: 341- 345.

PEAKALL, D.B. & BART, J.R. (1983) Impacts of aerial application of insecticides on forest birds. *CRC crit. Rev. environ. Control*, **13**: 117-165.

PIEPER, G.R. & RICHMOND, C.E. (1976) Residues of trichlorfon and lauroyl trichlorfon in Douglas fir, Willow grass, aspen, foliage and in creek water after aerial application. *Bull. environ. Contam. Toxicol.*, **15**: 250-256.

POMPONI, M., GIACOBINI, E., & BRUFANI, M. (1990) Present state and future development of Alzheimer diseases. *Aging*, **2**(2): 125-153.

POOLE, D.C., SIMMON, V.F., & NEWELL, G.W. (1977) *In vitro* mutagenic activity of fourteen pesticides. *Toxicol. appl. Pharmacol.*, **41**: 196 (Meeting abstract).

POPE, A.M., HEAVNER, J.E., GUARNIERI, J.A., & KNOBLOCH, C.P. (1986) Trichlorfon-induced congenital cerebellar hypoplasia in neonatal pigs. *J. Am. Vet. Med. Assoc.*, **189**: 781-783.

RASMUSSEN, F., BASSE, A., KRAUL, I., & DALGAARD-MIKKELSEN, Sr (1978) Inhibition of cholinesterase activity in blood from pregnant sows and hypoplasia of cerebellum in their piglets after oral application of metrifonate (neguvon(r) vet). In: *Nord. Vet. Congress Abo, July 1978.*

REINER, E., KRAUTHACKER, B. SIMEON, V., & SKRINJARIC-SPOLIJAR, M. (1975) Mechanism of inhibition *in vitro* of mammalian acetyl-cholinesterase and cholinesterase in solutions of *O,O*-dimethyl-2,2,2-trichloro-1-hydroxyethyl phosphonate (trichlorphon). *Biochem. Pharmacol.*, **24**: 717-722.

REISS, C.S., HERRMAN, J.M., & HOPKINS, R.E., II (1987) Effect of antihelminthic treatment on the immune response of mice. *Lab. anim. Sci.*, **37**: 773-775.

RICCIO, E., SHEPHERD, G., POMEROY, A., MORTELMANS, K., & WATERS, M.D. (1981) Comparative studies between the *S. cerevisiae* D3 and D7 assays of eleven pesticides. *Environ. Mutagen.*, **3**: 327 (Meeting abstract).

ROBBINS, W.E., HOPKINS, T.L., & EDDY, G.W. (1956) The metabolism of ^{32}P-labeled Bayer L13/59 in a cow. *J. econ. Entomol.*, **49**: 801-806.

ROBERTS, D. (1975) The effect of pesticides on byssus formation in the common mussel, *Mytilus edulis*. *Environ. Pollut.*, **8**: 241-254.

ROSENKRANZ, H.S. & ROSENKRANZ, S. (1972) Reaction of DNA with phosphoric acid esters: Gasoline additives and insecticides. *Experientia (Basel)*, **28**: 386-387.

RYAZANOVA, R.A. & GAFUROVA, T.V. (1980) [Mutagenic action of a binary mixture of the pesticides chlorophos and zineb.] *Gig. i Sanit.*, **1**: 80-81 (in Russian).

RYBAK, M. (1973) Effect of phosclor administered in water on the ontogenetic development of white rats and their offsprings. *Rocz. Panstw. Zakl. Hig.*, **24**: 465-475.

SALAMA, A.M., MOSTAFA, I.Y., & EL-ZAWAHRY, Y.A. (1975) Insecticides and soil microorganisms: (III) Fate of C-14 labeled Dipterex as affected by two nodule-forming *Rhizobium spp*. and roots of their respective leguminous host plants. *Acta biol. Acad. Sci. Hung.*, **26**: 1-7.

SASAKI, M., SUGIMURA, K., YOSHIDA, M., & ABE, S. (1980) Cytogenetic effects of 60 chemicals on cultured human and Chinese hamster cells. *Senshokutai*, **20**: 574-584.

SCHAFER, E.W. (1972) The acute oral toxicity of 369 pesticidal, pharmaceutical and other chemicals to wild birds. *Toxicol. appl. Pharmacol.*, **21**: 315-330.

SCHAFER, E.W., Jr, BOWLES, W.A. J, & HURLBUT, J. (1983) The acute oral toxicity, repellency, and hazard potential of 998 chemicals to one or more species of wild and domestic birds. *Arch. environ. Contam. Toxicol.*, **12**: 355-382.

SCHEUFLER, H. (1975) Effect of relatively high doses of dimethoate and trichlorfon on the embryogenesis of laboratory mice. *Biol. Rundsch.*, **13**: 238-240.

SCHIEMANN, S. (1975) Mutagenic effect of trichlorfon on the mouse, with special regard to the dominant lethal tests. *Wiss. Z. Martin-Luther-Univ. Halle-Wittenberg Math Naturwiss. R.*, **24**: 85-86.

SCHLINKE, J.C. & PALMER, J.S. (1973) Combined effects of phenothiazine and organophosphate insecticides in cattle. *J. Am. Vet. Med. Assoc.*, **163**: 756-758.

SCHULTEN, H.-R. & SUN, S.-E. (1981) Field desorption mass spectrometry of standard organophosphorus pesticides and their identification in waste water. *Int. J. environ. anal. Chem.*, **10**: 247- 264.

SERGEANT, D.B. & ZITKO, V. (1979) *The determination of trichlorfon, dichlorvos, fenitrothion and phosphamidon in water*, pp. 1-12 (Can. Fish Mars. Tech. Rep, 886).

SHIMAMOTO, K. & HATTORI, K. (1965) Effects of chronic feeding of the organic phosphorus compounds on the tissue cholinesterase in rats. *Acta med. Univ. Kyoto*, **39**: 128-137.

SHIRAISHI, S., GOTO, I., YAMASHITA, Y., OHNISHI, A., & NAGAO, H. (1977) [Dipterex polyneuropathy.] *Shinkei Naika*, **6**: 34-38 (in Japanese).

SHIRAISHI, S., INOUE, N., & MURAI, Y. (1982) Dipterex poisoning. *J. UOEH.*, **4**: 177-183.

SHIRAISHI, S., INOUE, N., MURAI, Y., ONISHI, A., & NODA, S. (1983) Dipterex (Trichlorfon) poisoning - clinical and pathological studies in human and monkeys. *J. UOEH.*, **5**(Suppl.): 125-132.

SHIRASU, Y., MORIYA, M., KATO, K., FURUHASHI, A., & KADA, T. (1976) Mutagenicity screening of pesticides in the microbial system. *Mutat. Res.*, **40**: 19-30.

SHIRASU, Y., MORIYA, M., KATO, K., TEZUKA, H., TERAMOTO, S., OHTA, T., & INOUE, T. (1982) Mutagenicity screening studies on pesticides. In: *Environmental mutagens and carcinogens*, Tokyo, University of Tokyo Press, pp. 331-335.

SILVESTRI, G.R., HIMES, J.A., & EDDS, G.T. (1975a) Repeated oral administration of coumaphos in sheep: effects on erythrocyte acetylcholinesterase and other constituents. *Am. J. Vet. Res.*, **36**: 283-287.

SILVESTRI, G.R., HIMES, J.A., & EDDS, G.T. (1975b) Repeated oral administration of coumaphos in sheep: interactions of coumaphos with bishydroxycoumarin, trichlorfon, and phenobarbital sodium. *Am. J. Vet. Res.*, **36**: 289-292.

SIMMON, V.F. (1979) In vitro *microbiological mutagenicity and unscheduled DNA synthesis studies of eighteen pesticides*, Research Triangle Park, North Carolina, US Environmental Protection Agency, pp. 79-81, 87, 111 (EPA-600/1-79-041).

SINGH, O. & AGARWAL, R.A. (1979) Effects on certain carbamate and organophosphorus pesticides on isolated organs of *Pila globosa* (Gastropoda). *Toxicol. appl. Pharmacol.*, **50**: 485-492.

SINGH, O. & AGARWAL, R.A. (1981) Toxicity of certain pesticides to two economic species of snails in northern India. *J. econ. Entomol.*, **74**: 568-571.

SISSONS, D.J. & TELLING, G.M. (1970) Rapid procedure for the determination of organophosphorus insecticide residues in vegetables. II. A screening procedure for water soluble insecticides. *J. Chromatogr.*, **48**: 468-477.

SLOTT, V. & ECOBICHON, D.J. (1984) An acute and subacute neurotoxicity assessment of trichlorfon. *Can. J. Physiol. Pharmacol.*, **62**: 513-518.

SNELLEN, W.M. (1981) Therapeutic properties of metrifonate. *Acta pharmacol. toxicol.*, **49**(Suppl.5): 114-117.

SOLIMAN, M.S., EL-MISSERY, A.G., ABDELMESSIH, M.S., FAYAD, M.E., & BASSILI, W.R. (1984) The effect of diazinon and neguvon on the liver of experimentally intoxicated mice. *J. Egypt. Soc. Parisitol.*, **14**: 557-562.

SPEHAR, R.L., LEMKE, A.E., PICKERING, Q.H., ROUSH, T.H., RUSSO, R.C., & YOUNT, J.D. (1981) Effects of pollution on freshwater fish. *J. Water Pollut. Control. Fed.*, **53**: 1028-1076.

SPICER, E.J.F. & URWIN, C. (1971) *Pathology report of Bay 15922 generation experiment in rats* (Unpublished report submitted to WHO by Farbenfabriken Bayer AG, Germany).

STAN, H.J. (1977) [Detection of organophosphorous pesticide residues in food at the ppb level with open tubular column gas chromatography- mass spectrometry.] *Z. Lebensm. Unters. Forsch.*, **164**: 153-159 (in German).

STAN, H.J., ABRAHAM, B., JUNG, J., KELLERT, M., & STEINLAND, K. (1977) [Detection of organophosphorus insecticides by gas chromatography/mass spectrometry.] *Fresenius Z. anal. Chem.*, **287**: 271-285 (in German).

STAPLES, R.E. & GOULDING, E.H. (1979) Dipterex teratogenicity in the rat, hamster and mouse when given by gavage. *Environ. Health Perspect.*, **30**: 105-113.

STAPLES, R.E., KELLAM, R.G., & HASEMAN, J.K. (1976) Developmental toxicity in the rat after ingestion or gavage of organophosphate pesticides (dipterex, imidan) during pregnancy. *Environ. Health Perspect.*, **13**: 133-140.

STOBWASSER, H. & KIRCHHOFF, J. (1968) [Insecticide residues on lettuce and spinach in outdoor and greenhouse cultivation.] *Qual. Plant Mater. Veg.*, **15**: 273-279 (in German).

SUGIYAMA, H. & SHIGEMATSU, H. (1969) Enzymic dehydrochlorination of trichlorfon by the digestive juice of the silkworm. *Bombyx mori. Botyu-Kagaku*, **34**: 79-85.

SUNDARAM, K.M.S. & VARTY, I.W. (1989) Distribution and persistence of trichlorfon in a forest environment. *J. Environ. Sci. Health*, **B 24**(6): 647-659.

SZALONTAI, G. (1976) High-performance liquid chromatography of organophosphorus insecticides. *J. Chromatogr.*, **124**: 9-16.

SZUBARTOWSKA, E. (1983) Peripheral blood picture in rabbits poisoned by the pesticide trichlorfon. *Folia biol.*, **31**: 407-418.

SZUBARTOWSKA, E. & GROMYSZ-KALKOWSKA, K. (1986) Differences between breeds of rabbits in their susceptibility to the effect of foschlor. *Comp. Biochem. Physiol.*, **85C**: 33-40.

TAKASE, I., NAKAHARA, T., YOSHIMOTO, Y., & NAKAMURA, H. (1972) [Determination of residues of trichlorfon and its metabolites in plants, milk, chicken, and fish by gas chromatography.] *Botyu-Kagaku*, **37**: 142-148 (in Japanese).

TAYLOR, P. (1980) Anticholinesterase agents. In: Gilman, A.G., Goodman, L.S. & Gilman, A., ed. *The pharmacological basis of therapeutics*, 6th ed., New York, MacMillan Publishing Co., pp. 100-119.

TEICHMANN, B. & HAUSCHILD, F. (1978) [Test of *O,O*-dimethyl(1-hydroxy-2,2,2-trichloro-ethyl)phosphonate (Trichlorfon) for carginogenic activity in mice by oral (oesophageal-gastric intubation), intraperitoneal and dermal application.] *Arch. Geschwulstforsch*, **48**: 301-307 (in German).

TEICHMANN, B. & SCHMIDT, A. (1978) [Test of *O,O*-dimethyl(1-hydroxy-2,2,2-trichloro-ethyl)phosphonate(Trichlorfon) for carcinogenic activity in Syrian golden hamsters (*Mesocricetus auratus* Waterhouse) by intraperitoneal administration.] *Arch. Geschwulst-forsch*, **48**: 718-721 (in German).

TEICHMANN, B., HAUSCHILD, F., & ECKELMANN, A. (1978) [Test of *O,O*-dimethyl (1-hydroxy-2,2,2-trichloroethyl)phosphonate (Trichlorofon) for carcinogenic activity in rats by oral (oesophageal-gastric intubation) and intraperitoneal administration.] *Arch. Geschwulstforsch.*, **48**: 112-119, (in German).

TELEUGALIEV, T.M. (1977) [Veterinary hygienic study of fish poisoned with trichlorfon.] *Vestn. S-kh. Nauki Kaz.*, **20**: 75-77 (in Russian).

THYSSEN, J. (1981) *L 13/59 (Dipterex active ingredient) tests for skin and eye irritation*, Wuppertal-Elberfeld, Bayer AG, Institute of Toxicology, (Proprietary report submitted to WHO by Bayer AG, Germany).

TREFILOV, V.N., FAEDMAN, I.S., & BORISOVA, E.P. (1971) [Contamination of working clothes and skin of workers engaged in the production of metaphos and chlorophos.] *Gig. Tr. prof. Zabol.*, **15**: 51-53 (in Russian).

TRINH VAN BAO, SZABO, I., RUZICSKA, P., & CZEIZEL, A. (1974) Chromosome aberrations in patients suffering acute organic phosphate insecticide intoxication. *Humangenetik*, **24**: 33-57.

TSUMUKI, H., SAITO, T., MIYATA, T., & IYATOMI, K. (1970) Acute and subacute toxicity of organophosphorus insecticides to mammals. In: O'Brien, R.D. & Yamamoto, I., ed. *Biochemical toxicology of insecticides*, New York, London, Academic Press, pp. 65-73.

TSVETKOVA, T.S., PENEVA, V., & GRIGOROVA, D. (1981) [Residual amount of pesticides in honey.] *Vet. Med. Nauki*, **18**: 93-98 (in Russian).

UMEHARA, F., FUKUOKA, T., MINAUCHI, Y., OSAME, M., & IGATA, A. (1982) A case of dipterex poisoning. A histopathological study of peripheral nerves. *Clin. Neurol.*, **22**: 990-996.

US NTP (1989) *NTP technical report on the toxicology and carcinogenesis studies of dichlorvos (CAS No: 62-73-7) in F344/N rats and B6C3F$_1$ mice (gavage studies)*, Research Triangle Park, North Carolina, National Toxicology Program (NTP TR 342).

VALENCIA, R. (1977) Mutagenesis screening of pesticides using drosophia (Contract No. 68-01-2474), Madison, Wisconsin, WARF Institute, Inc.

VAN MIDDELEM, C.H., HABECK, D.H., & STRAYER, J.R. (1972) Residues on ryegrass following preplant or postemergence applications of four insecticides for mole cricket control. *J. econ. Entmol.*, **65**: 495-497.

VASILESCU, C., ALEXIANU, M., & DAN, A. (1984) Delayed neuropathy after organophosphorus insecticides (Dipterex) poisoning: a clinical, electrophysiological, and nerve biopsy study. *J. Neurol. Neurosurg. Psychiatry.*, **47**: 543-548.

VILCEANU, R., SCHULZ, P., DRAGHICI, R., & SOIMU, P. (1973) [Gas chromatography of (1-hydroxy-2,2,2-trichlorethyl)-phosphonic acid esters.] *J. Chromatogr.*, **82**: 285-290 (in German).

VÖLKNER, W. (1987) L 13/59 (Trichlorfon) - *Sister chromatid exchanges (SCEs) in Chinese hamster bone marrow cells,* Technical University of Darmstadt, Laboratory for Mutagenicity Testing (Proprietary report No. R 4079, submitted to WHO by Bayer AG, Germany).

WATERS, M.D., SIMMON, V.F., MITCHELL, A.D., JORGENSON, T.A., & VALENCIA, R. (1980) An overview of short-term tests for the mutagenic and carcinogenic potential of pesticides. *J. environ. Sci. Health*, **B15**: 867-906.

WATERS, M.D., NESNOW, S., SIMMON, A.D., MITCHELL, T.A., JORGENSON, T.A., & VALENCIA, R. (1981) Pesticides: mutagenic and carcinogenic potential. In: Bandal, S.K., Golberg, L., & Leng, M.L., ed. *The pesticide chemist and modern toxicology*, Washington, DC, American Chemical Society, pp. 80-113 (ACS Symposium Series, No. 160).

WATERS, M.D., SANDHU, S.S., SIMMON, V.F., MORTELMANS, K.E., MITCHELL, A.D., JORGENSON, T.A., JONES, D.C.L., VALENCIA, R., & GARRET, N.E. (1982) Study of pesticide genotoxicity. *Basic Life Sci.*, **21**: 275-326.

WEGNER, D. (1970) [Bilarcil® Bay 2349 - Clinical experience 1960-1969.] (Unpublished report submitted to WHO by Farbenfabriken Bayer AG, Germany.) (in German).

WELLBORN, T.L., Jr (1969) The toxicity of nine therapeutic and herbicidal compounds to striped bass. *Prog. Fish Cult.*, **31**: 27-32.

WENDA-ROZEWICKA, L. (1983) Morphometric studies of male gonads from mice receiving insecticides (Metox-30, Sadofos-30, and Foschlor-50). *Folia biol.*, **32**: 23-34.

WHO (1985) *The control of schistosomiasis: Report of a WHO expert committee*, Geneva, World Health Organization, pp. 113 (Technical Report Series, No. 728).

WHO (1986) *Environmental Health Criteria 63: Organophosphorus insecticides: A general introduction*, Geneva, World Health Organization, pp. 181.

WHO (1989) *Environmental Health Criteria 79: Dichlorvos*, Geneva, World Health Organization, pp. 157.

WHO (1990) *The WHO recommended classification of pesticides by hazard and guidelines to classification 1990-1991*, Geneva, World Health Organization, pp. 39 (Unpublished document WHO/PCS/90.1 Rev.1).

WHO/FAO (1977) *Data sheets on pesticides, No. 27: Trichlorfon*, Geneva, World Health Organization, pp. 9 (VBC/DS/77.28).

WILD, D. (1975) Mutagenicity studies on organophosphorus insecticides. *Mutat. Res.*, **32**: 133-150.

WILKINS, H.A. & MOORE, P.J. (1987) Comparative trials of regimes for the treatment of urinary schistomiasis in the Gambia. *J. trop. Med. Hyg.*, **90**: 83-92.

WILLIAMS, M.W., FUYAT, H.N., & FITZHUGH, O.G. (1959) The subacute toxicity of four organic phosphates to dogs. *Toxicol. appl. Pharmacol.*, **1**: 1-7.

WINTERLIN, W., WALKER, G., & FRANK, H. (1968) Detection of cholinesterase-inhibiting pesticides following separation on thin-layer chromatograms. *J. agric. food Chem.*, **16**: 808-812.

WOODWARD, D.F. & MAUCK, W.L. (1980) Toxicity of five forest insecticides to cutthroat trout *Salmo clarki* and two species of aquatic invertebrates. *Bull. environ. Contam. Toxicol.*, **25**: 846-853.

WRIGHT, A.S., HUTSON, D.H., & WOODER, A.F. (1979) The chemical and biochemical reactivity of dichlorvos. *Arch. Toxicol.*, **42**: 1-18.

YAKOUB (1990) *A rational approach to the treatment of Schistosoma haematobium infection with metrifonate - clinical and pharmacological studies*, Stockholm, Karolinska Institute, (Dissertation).

YASHIKI, M., KOJIMA, T., & UNE, I. (1982) [Determination of Dipterex in biological materials by gas chromatography and gas chromatography- mass spectrometry and the analysis of the distribution of Dipterex in a case of fatal poisoning.] *Nippon Hoigaku Zasshi*, **36**: 426-430 (in Japanese).

YASHIKI, M., CHIKASUE, F., MIYAZAKI, T., KOJIMA, T., & OHTANI, M. (1988) [Gas chromatographic and gas chromatographic-mass spectrometric determination of trichlorfon in biological fluids collected in a fatal dipterex poisoning.] *Nippon Hoigaku Zasshi*, **42**: 94-98 (in Japanese, with English summary).

YONOVA, I. & ZHECHEVA, G. (1974) [Residues of sevin, trichlorfon and imidan in the meat of pig treated for ectoparasites.] *Vet. Med. Nauki*, **11**: 28-34 (in Russian).

YÜKSEKISIK, N. (1973) Kinetic study of the rearrangement of *O,O*- dialkyl 2,2,2-tricholoro-1-hydroxyethylphosphonates. *Commun. Fac. Sci. Univ. Ankara Ser.*, **B 20**: 49-62.

YUROVSKAYA, E.M. & ZHULINSKAYA, V.A. (1974) [Behavior of organophosphorous insecticides in the soil.] *Khim. Sel'sk. Khoz.*, **12**: 358-361 (in Russian).

ZAKHAROV, B.N. (1980) [Migration of trichlorfon in nature.] *Gig. i Sanit.*, **45**: 62-63 (in Russian).

ZAYED, S.M.A.D., MOSTAFA, I.Y., & HASSAN, A. (1965) Metabolism of organophosphorus insecticides. (VII) Transformation of ^{32}P-labeled Dipterex through microorganisms. *Arch. Mikrobiol.*, **51**: 118-121.

ZELINSKIY, M.I. (1974) [Toxicity of trichlorfon and its effect on the quality of meat.] *Vestn. S-kh. Nauki Kaz.*, **17**(10): 66-68 (in Russian).

ZINKL, J.G., HENNY, C.J., & DEWEESE, L.R. (1977) Brain cholinesterase activities of birds from forests sprayed with trichlorfon (Dylox) and carbaryl (Sevin-4-oil). *Bull. environ. Contam. Toxicol.*, **17**: 379-386.

ZWEIG, G. & SHERMA, J. (1972) Dylox. In: *Analytical methods for pesticides and plant growth regulators,* New York, London, Academic Press, Vol. 6, pp. 387-392.

ANNEX I. TREATMENT OF ORGANOPHOSPHATE INSECTICIDE POISONING IN MAN

(From EHC 63: Organophosphorus Insecticides - A General Introduction)

All cases of organophosphorus poisoning should be dealt with as an emergency and the patient sent to hospital as quickly as possible. Although symptoms may develop rapidly, delay in onset or a steady increase in severity may be seen up to 48 h after ingestion of some formulated organophosphorus insecticides.

Extensive descriptions of treatment of poisoning by organophosphorus insecticides are given in several major references (Kagan, 1977; Taylor, 1980; UK DHSS, 1983; Plestina, 1984) and will also be included in the IPCS Health and Safety Guides to be prepared for selected organophosphorus insecticides.

The treatment is based on:

(a) minimizing the absorption;
(b) general supportive treatment; and
(c) specific pharmacological treatment.

I.1 Minimizing the absorption

When dermal exposure occurs, decontamination procedures include removal of contaminated clothes and washing of the skin with alkaline soap or with a sodium bicarbonate solution. Particular care should be taken in cleaning the skin area where venepuncture is performed. Blood might be contaminated with direct-acting organophosphorus esters and, therefore, inaccurate measures of ChE inhibition might result. Extensive eye irrigation with water or saline should also be performed. In the case of ingestion, vomiting might be induced, if the patient is conscious, by the administration of ipecacuanha syrup (10-30 ml) followed by 200 ml water. This treatment is, however, contraindicated in the case of pesticides dissolved in hydrocarbon solvents. Gastric lavage (with addition of bicarbonate solution or activated charcoal) can also be performed, particularly in unconscious patients, taking care to prevent aspiration of fluids into the lungs (i.e., only after a tracheal tube has been put into place).

The volume of fluid introduced into the stomach should be recorded and samples of gastric lavage frozen and stored for subsequent chemical analysis. If the formulation of the pesticide involved is available, it should also be stored for further analysis (i.e., detection of toxicologically relevant impurities). A purgative can be administered to remove the ingested compound.

I.2 General supportive treatment

Artificial respiration (via a tracheal tube) should be started at the first sign of respiratory failure and maintained for as long as necessary.

Cautious administration of fluids is advised, as well as general supportive and symptomatic pharmacological treatment and absolute rest.

I.3 Specific pharmacological treatment

I.3.1 Atropine

Atropine should be given, beginning with 2 mg iv and given at 15-30-min intervals. The dose and the frequency of atropine treatment varies from case to case, but should maintain the patient fully atropinized (dilated pupils, dry mouth, skin flushing, etc.). Continuous infusion of atropine may be necessary in extreme cases and total daily doses up to several hundred mg may be necessary during the first few days of treatment.

I.3.2 Oxime reactivators

Cholinesterase reactivators (e.g., pralidoxime, obidoxime) specifically restore AChE activity inhibited by organophosphates. This is not the case with enzymes inhibited by carbamates. The treatment should begin as soon as possible, because oximes are not effective on "aged" phosphorylated ChEs. However, if absorption, distribution, and metabolism are thought to be delayed for any reasons, oximes can be administered for several days after intoxication. Effective treatment with oximes reduces the required dose of atropine. Pralidoxime is the most widely available oxime. A dose of 1 g pralidoxime can be given either im or iv and repeated

2-3 times per day or, in extreme cases, more often. If possible, blood samples should be taken for AChE determinations before and during treatment. Skin should be carefully cleansed before sampling. Results of the assays should influence the decision whether to continue oxime therapy after the first 2 days.

There are indications that oxime therapy may possibly have beneficial effects on CNS-derived symptoms.

I.3.3 Diazepam

Diazepam should be included in the therapy of all but the mildest cases. Besides relieving anxiety, it appears to counteract some aspects of CNS-derived symptoms that are not affected by atropine. Doses of 10 mg sc or iv are appropriate and may be repeated as required (Vale & Scott, 1974). Other centrally acting drugs and drugs that may depress respiration are not recommended in the absence of artificial respiration procedures.

I.3.4 Notes on the recommended treatment

I.3.4.1 Effects of atropine and oxime

The combined effect far exceeds the benefit of either drug singly.

I.3.4.2 Response to atropine

The response of the eye pupil may be unreliable in cases of organophosphorus poisoning. A flushed skin and drying of secretions are the best guide to the effectiveness of atropinization. Although repeated dosing may well be necessary, excessive doses at any one time may cause toxic side-effects. Pulse-rate should not exceed 120/min.

I.3.4.3 Persistence of treatment

Some organophosphorus pesticides are very lipophilic and may be taken into, and then released from, fat depots over a period of many days. It is therefore quite incorrect to abandon oxime treatment after 1-2 days on the supposition that all inhibited enzyme will be aged. Ecobichon et al. (1977) noted prompt improvement in both condition and blood-ChEs in response to pralidoxime given on the 11th-15th days after major symptoms of poisoning appeared due to extended exposure to fenitrothion (a dimethyl phosphate with a short half-life for aging of inhibited AChE).

I.3.4.4 Dosage of atropine and oxime

The recommended doses above pertain to exposures, usually for an occupational setting, but, in the case of very severe exposure or massive ingestion (accidental or deliberate), the therapeutic doses may be extended considerably. Warriner et al. (1977) reported the case of a patient who drank a large quantity of dicrotophos, in error, while drunk. Therapeutic dosages were progressively increased up to 6 mg atropine iv every 15 min together with continuous iv infusion of pralidoxime chloride at 0.5 g/h for 72 h, from days 3 to 6 after intoxication. After considerable improvement, the patient relapsed and further aggressive therapy was given at a declining rate from days 10 to 16 (atropine) and to day 23 (oxime), respectively. In total, 92 g of pralidoxime chloride and 3912 mg of atropine were given and the patient was discharged on the thirty-third day with no apparent sequelae.

References to Annex I.

ECOBICHON, D.J., OZERE, R.L., REID, E., & CROCKER, J.F.S (1977) Acute fenitrothion poisoning. *Can. Med. Assoc. J.*, **116**: 377-379.

KAGAN, JU.S. (1977) [*Toxicology of organophosphorus pesticides*], Moscow, Meditsina, pp. 111-121, 219-233, 260-269 (in Russian).

PLESTINA, R. (1984) *Prevention, diagnosis, and treatment of insecticide poisoning*, Geneva, World Health Organization (Unpublished document VBC/84.889).

TAYLOR, P. (1980) Anticholinesterase agents. In: Goodman, L.S. & Gilman, A., ed. *The pharmacological basis of therapeutics*, 6th ed., New York, Macmillan Publishing Company, pp. 100-119.

UK DHSS (1983) *Pesticide poisoning: notes for the guidance of medical practitioners*, London, United Kingdom Department of Health and Social Security, pp. 41-47.

VALE, J.A. & SCOTT, G.W. (1974) Organophosphorus poisoning. *Guy's Hosp. Rep.*, **123**: 13-25.

WARRINER, R.A., III, NIES, A.S., & HAYES, W.J., Jr (1977) Severe organophosphate poisoning complicated by alcohol and terpentine ingestion. *Arch. environ. Health*, **32**: 203-205.

ANNEX II. NO-OBSERVED-EFFECT LEVELS (NOELS) IN ANIMALS TREATED WITH TRICHLORFON

Annex II, No-observed-effect levels (NOELS) in animals treated with trichlorfon

Animal (strain)	Exposure[a]	NOEL (paramater)	Reference
Rat	16 weeks	100 mg/kg diet (ChE)	Doull & Dubois (1956)
Dog	12 weeks	200 mg/kg diet (plasma, Er-ChE)	Williams et al. (1959)
Rat	6h/day over 3 weeks	12.7 mg/m^3 by inhalation (plasma, Er, brain ChE)	Kimmerle (1975b)
Beagle dog	12 months	250 mg/kg diet (ChE)	Doull et al. (1962a)
Beagle dog	4 years	50 mg/kg diet (ChE)	Löser (1970)
Rhesus monkey	26 weeks	0.2 mg/kg body weight oral intubation (Er-ChE)	Hoffmann et al. (1988)
CD-1 mouse	90 weeks	100 mg/kg diet (ChE) 1000 mg/kg diet (tumour incidence)	Machemer (1981)
CD-1 mouse	104 weeks	2700 mg/kg diet (tumorigenicity)	Hayes (1988)

Annex II. (continued)

Animal (strain)	Exposure[a]	NOEL (paramater)	Reference
Sprague-Dawley rat	17 months (m) 24 months (f)	250 mg/kg diet (ChE, survival, spermatogenesis, ovarian changes) 50 mg/kg diet (mammary tumours)	Doull et al. (1962b)
Sprague-Dawley rat	18 months	200 mg/kg diet (ovarian changes)	Doull et al. (1965)
Long-Evans rat	24 months	500 mg/kg diet (ChE) 1000 mg/kg diet (tumorigenicity)	Lorke & Löser (1966); Grundmann & Hobik (1966)
Rat	twice/week for 90 weeks	22 mg/kg body weight by gavage (incidence of tumours)	Teichmann et al. (1978)
Fischer 344 rat	105 weeks	100 mg/kg diet (morphological parameters)	Hayes (1989)
Rhesus monkey	6 days/week for 10 years	0.2 mg/kg body weight oral intubation (brain-ChE)	Griffin (1988)

Annex II. (continued)

AB/Jena mouse	twice/week for 75 weeks	28.2 mg/body weight ip injection (incidence of tumours)	Teichmann & Hauschild (1978)
Rat	twice/week for 90 weeks	12.0 mg/kg body weight ip injection (incidence of tumours)	Teichmann et al. (1978)
Syrian Golden hamster	once/week for 90 weeks	20 mg/kg body weight ip injection (incidence of tumours)	Teichmann & Schmidt (1978)
AB/Jena mouse	twice/week for 75 weeks	0.25 ml of 1% solution in acetone dermal administration (incidence of tumours)	Teichmann & Hauschild (1978)

[a] m = male.
f = female.

RESUME ET EVALUATION, CONCLUSIONS ET RECOMMANDATIONS

1. Résumé et évaluation

1.1 Exposition

Le trichlorfon est un insecticide organophosphoré utilisé depuis le début des années 1950. En agriculture, on l'emploie principalement contre les ravageurs des cultures de plein champ et des vergers. On l'utilise également comme insecticide en forêt et pour débarrasser des animaux domestiques de leurs parasites. Sous le nom de métrifonate, il est utilisé pour traiter l'infestation humaine à *Schistosoma haematobium*. Il agit en libérant lentement du dichlorvos. Le trichlorfon est commercialisé sous forme de concentré émulsionnable, de poudre dispersable, de poudre pour poudrage, de granulés, de solution et de concentré à très bas volume.

Peu après l'épandage, la concentration atmosphérique du trichlorfon peut atteindre 0,1 mg/m^3 mais cette valeur diminue rapidement pour tomber à moins de 0,01 mg/m^3 en quelques jours. Les eaux de ruissellement provenant des zones traitées peuvent contenir des concentrations de trichlorfon atteignant 50 μg/litre, mais la teneur des eaux de surface est généralement beaucoup faible et diminue rapidement.

Le trichlorfon se décompose rapidement dans le sol et sa concentration y devient généralement négligeable dans le mois qui suit l'épandage. Il est relativement stable dans l'eau aux pH inférieurs à 5,5. A pH plus élevé, il se transforme de dichlorvos. Les microorganismes et les plantes métabolisent probablement le trichlorfon mais son mode d'élimination principal est l'hydrolyse abiotique.

A quelques exceptions près, la concentration de trichlorfon sur les récoltes est inférieure à 10 mg/kg dans le jour qui suit l'épandage et tombe en-dessous de 0,1 mg/kg une quinzaine jours après.

Le lait des vaches que l'on a traitées au trichlorfon pour les débarrasser de leur vermine peut contenir des résidus atteignant 1,2 mg/litre deux heures après l'application, mais cette valeur tombe en-dessous de 0,1 mg/litre dans les 24 heures. On n'a pas constaté la présence de concentrations importantes de trichlorfon dans la viande des animaux traités. Dans les oeufs de poules traitées on a mesuré des concentrations de 0,05 mg/kg.

1.2 Absorption, métabolisme et excrétion

Le trichlorfon est rapidement absorbé par l'ensemble des voies d'exposition (orale, dermique, respiratoire) et il se répartit rapidement dans les tissus de l'organisme. Le taux sanguin passe par un maximum au bout d'une à deux heures, le produit disparaissant presque totalement du courant sanguin au bout 1,5 à 4 heures. La demi-vie biologique du trichlorfon dans le sang des mammifères a été estimée à environ 30 minutes.

Dans l'eau, les liquides biologiques et les tissus, à des valeurs du pH supérieures à 5,5 le trichlorfon subit une transformation en dichlorvos (phosphate de 2,2-dichlorovinyle et de diméthyle) par déshydrochloration. C'est le dichlorvos qui constitue le principe actif antichlolinestérasique. Les principales voies de dégradation sont la déméthylation, la coupure de la liaison phosphore-carbone et l'hydrolyse de l'ester via le dichlorvos. Les principaux métabolites du trichlorfon que l'on trouve *in vivo* sont le déméthyltrichlorfon, le déméthyldichlorvos, l'hydrogénophosphate de diméthyle, l'hydrogénophosphate de méthyle l'acide phosphorique et de trichloréthanol. Ce dernier métabolite se retrouve dans l'urine, conjugué sous forme de glucuronide.

Le trichlorfon et ses métabolites sont principalement éliminés par voie urinaire. Des études effectuées avec du trichlorfon radiomarqué (^{14}C-méthyl et ^{32}P) ont montré que la majeure partie du produit s'éliminait sous la forme de dérivés hydrosolubles et une faible fraction sous la forme de dérivés solubles dans le chloroforme. Environ 66 à 70 % des produits hydrosolubles apparaissent dans l'urine dans les 12 heures, 24 % du produit radiomarqué au niveau du groupement méthyl étant éliminés dans l'air expiré sous forme de dioxyde de carbone (CO_2). Après avoir traité des vaches soit par administration orale soit par voie cutanée, on a retrouvé dans leur lait de faibles quantités de trichlorfon et de ses métabolites.

1.3 Effets sur les êtres vivants dans leur milieu naturel

Le trichlorfon est modérément toxique pour les poissons (les valeurs de la CL_{50} à 96 heures vont de 0,45 mg/litre à 51 mg/litre) et modérément à fortement toxique pour les arthropodes aquatiques (valeur de la CL_{50} à 48 et 96 heures comprises en entre 0,75 μg/litre et 7800 μg/litre). Toutefois les concentrations dont il est fait état dans les eaux superficielles après épandage dans des forêts à la dose de 6kg/ha, sont inférieures à ces valeurs. Il s'en suit qu'en utilisation normale, le trichlorfon n'aura guère d'effets sur les organismes aquatiques car les autres types d'organismes tels que les mollusques et les microorganismes sont moins sensibles que les arthropodes. Les valeurs de la DL_{50} tirées d'études en laboratoire se situent entre 40 et 180 mg/kg et montrent donc que le trichlorfon est modérément toxique pour les oiseaux. Toutefois des études menées sur le terrain après épandage de trichlorfon par voie aérienne sur des forêts, n'ont révélé aucun effet sur l'effectif, la formation de couples, le nichage ou la mortalité des oiseaux chanteurs. La diminution du chant et l'accroissement de l'activité trophique qui ont été constatés sont peut-être la conséquence d'une réduction du nombre de proies. Rien n'indique que le trichlorfon puisse avoir un effet nocif sur la faune terrestre, à part les arthropodes. On ne possède aucune donnée au sujet des effets de cet insecticide sur les arthropodes utiles.

1.4 Effets sur les animaux d'expérience et sur les systèmes d'épreuves in vitro

Le trichlorfon est un insecticide modérément toxique pour les animaux d'expérience. Chez l'animal de laboratoire, les valeurs de la DL_{50} pour le trichlorfon technique s'étagent de 400 à 800 mg/kg de poids corporel et pour le rat, la DL_{50} cutanée dépasse 2000 mg/kg de poids corporel.

L'intoxication par le trichlorfon offre le tableau clinique habituel de l'atteinte cholinergique due aux organophosphorés et qui résulte d'une accumulation d'acétylcholine au niveau des terminaisons nerveuses.

On a montré que le trichlorfon technique était modérément irritant pour la conjonctive chez le rat, aucun effet de ce genre n'ayant été noté lors de tests cutanés sur des lapins. Sa capacité de sensibilisation cutanée a été mise en évidence chez le cobaye.

Des études de toxicité par voie orale de brève durée ont été effectuées sur des rats, des chiens, des singes, des lapins et des cobayes. Lors d'une étude de 16 semaines sur des rats, de 4 ans sur des chiens et de 26 semaines sur des singes, on a fixé respectivement à 100 mg/kg de nourriture, 5' mg/kg de nourriture et 0,2 mg/kg de nourriture la dose sans effet observé (sur la base de l'activité cholinestérasique, plasmatique, érythrocytaire ou cérébrale). En exposant par voie respiratoire des rats pendant trois semaines, on a obtenu une dose sans effet observé de 12,7 mg/m^3 en se basant sur l'inhibition de l'activité cholinestérasique du plasma, des érythrocytes et du cerveau. Des études de toxicité et de cancérogénicité à long terme ont été menées sur des souris, des rats, des singes et des hamsters à qui l'on a administré du trichlorfon par voie orale,intrapéritonéale ou percutanée. Après exposition par voie orale des souris et des rats à des doses de 30 mg/kg de poids corporel et de 400 mg/kg de nourriture respectivement, on a observé des anomalies au niveau des gonades. Lors d'une étude de 24 mois sur des rats et de 10 ans sur des singes, on a obtenu des doses sans effet observé respectivement égales à 50 mg/kg de nourriture et 0,2 mg/kg de poids corporel. Les données sont on dispose ne permettent pas de conclure que la substance est cancérogène après administration à des animaux de laboratoire pendant une longue période par diverses voies.

Dans les conditions physiologiques , le trichlorfon est susceptible d'alkyler l'ADN. Les tests de mutagénicité ont donné des résultats tantôt positifs tantôt négatifs. Il a peut que les effets observés soient imputables en tout ou partie au dichlorvos. La plupart des études de mutagénicité effectuées *in vitro* sur des bactéries ou des cellules mammaliennes ont donné des résultats positifs alors que rares sont les études *in vivo* qui ont donné de tels résultats.

L'expérimentation sur la souris, le rat et le hamster montre que le trichlorfon suscite une réaction tératogène chez le rat à des doses suffisantes pour être toxiques chez la mère. Après avoir administré à des rattes en cours de gestation une dose de 145 mg de trichlorfon par kg de nourriture, on a observé des malformations chez les foetus. Une dose de 400 mg/kg de poids corporel administrée par gavage à des hamsters a également été toxique pour les mères et a provoqué des effets tératogènes. La dose la plus faible administrée par gavage et ayant provoqué des effets tératogènes chez le rat était de 80 mg/kg de poids corporel. Au cours de la période de gestation, les effets produits présentent une spécificité chronologique. Cette étude a permis de fixer à 8 mg/kg la dose sans effet observé.

Des doses sans effet observé respectivement égales à 8 mg/kg et à 200 mg/kg de poids corporel ont été observées chez le rat et le hamster. Chez le porc et le cobaye, on a constaté une action tératogène sur le système nerveux central.

Cependant, aucun effet tératogène n'a été observé lors d'une étude de reproduction portant sur trois générations de rats, au cours de laquelle on a relevé des effets nocifs sur la fonction de reproduction. Dans cette étude, la dose sans effet observé était de 300 mg/kg de nourriture.

A très hautes doses, le trichlorfon produit des effets neurotoxiques chez l'animal.

Chez les mammifères, le métabolite actif est le dichlorvos, dont l'activité anticholinestérasique est au moins 100 fois plus forte que celle du trichlorfon.

1.5 *Effets sur l'homme*

Plusieurs cas d'intoxication aiguë délibérée (suicide) ou accidentelle se sont produits. L'intoxication présente une symptomatologie caractéristique de l'inhibition de la cholinestérase : épuisement, faiblesse, confusion, sueur et salivation profuses, douleurs abdominales, vomissements, myosis et spasmes musculaires. Dans les cas graves, l'intoxication entraîne la perte de conscience et des convulsions et la mort survient généralement par insuffisance respiratoire. Chez les victimes qui ont survécu à l'intoxication grâce à une intervention médicale, on a observé quelquefois, plusieurs semaines après l'exposition, une polyneuropathie retardée accompagnée d'une faiblesse des membres inférieurs. Dans les cas mortels, l'autopsie a révélé des foyers d'ischémie dans le cerveau, la moelle épinière et les ganglions végétatifs, ainsi que des lésions de la gaine de myéline dans la moelle épinière et les pédoncules cérébraux, avec des altérations dans la structure des axones des nerfs périphériques.

Les quelques cas d'intoxication d'origine professionnelle qui se sont produits, s'expliquent essentiellement par des négligences au niveau de la sécurité. L'exposition professionnelle sur les lieux de travail à des concentrations atmosphériques supérieures à 0,5 mg/m^3 a entraîné une réduction de la cholinestérase plasmatique et une altération du tracé électroencéphalographique. Toutefois ces anomalies ont complètement régressé à l'arrêt de l'exposition. Aucun cas de sensibilisation cutanée n'a été signalé.

Ce composé est très largement utilisé pour le traitement de la schistosomiase chez l'homme. L'administration d'une dose unique (7 à 12 mg/kg) entraîne une inhibition de la cholinestérase plasmatique et érythrocytaire à hauteur de 40-60 %, sans entraîner de symptômes cholinergiques. Toutefois, des symptômes légers ont été observés chez des malades qui avaient pris de ce produit à plusieurs reprises. A forte dose (24 mg/kg) on a observé de graves symptômes cholinergiques

2. Conclusions

- Le trichlorfon est un insecticide organophosphoré modérément toxique. Une intoxication grave peut survenir par suite d'une exposition excessive au produit lors de sa manipulation, de sa fabrication ou de son utilisation ou par suite d'une ingestion accidentelle ou délibérée.

- L'exposition au trichlorfon de la population générale résulte principalement de son utilisation en agriculture et en médecine vétérinaire et dans le traitement de la schistosomiase (bilharziose).

- Les quantités de trichlorfon qui sont absorbées sont très inférieures à la dose journalière administrable fixée par la FAO et l'OMS et ne devraient pas constituer une menace pour la santé publique.

- Si l'on adopte de bonnes méthodes de travail et, que l'on respecte les précautions d'hygiène et de sécurité, le trichlorfon n'est vraisemblablement pas dangereux pour les personnes qui sont exposées de par leur profession.

- Bien que le trichlorfon soit très toxique pour les arthropodes non visés, son utilisation n'entraîne guère d'effets nocifs sur la faune et la flore.

3. Recommandations

- Afin de préserver la santé et le bien-être des ouvriers et de la population en général, il importe de confier la manipulation et l'épandage du trichlorfon exclusivement à des personnes correctement encadrées et expérimentées, qui sauront appliquer les mesures de sécurité indispeurables et utiliser convenablement le produit.

- Des précautions sont à observer lors de la production, de la formulation, de l'utilisation en agriculture et du rejet du trichlorfon afin de contaminer le moins possible l'environnement et plus spécialement des eaux de surface.

- Les travailleurs qui sont régulièrement exposés au trichlorfon ainsi que les malades traités avec ce produit doivent subir des examens médicaux périodiques.

- Les doses d'emploi en agriculture devront rester faibles afin d'éviter la destruction des arthropodes non visés. L'insecticide ne devra jamais être épandu sur des étendues ou des cours d'eau.

RESUMEN Y EVALUACION, CONCLUSIONES Y RECOMENDACIONES

1. Resumen y evaluación

1.1 Exposición

El triclorfón es un insecticida organofosforado que lleva utilizándose desde principios de los años cincuenta. En agricultura sirve principalmente para combatir las plagas de insectos en los cultivos extensivos y en los frutales. Se utiliza asimismo para combatir los insectos de los bosques y los parásitos de los animales domésticos. Bajo la denominación de metrifonato, se emplea para tratar la infestación del hombre por *Schistosoma haematobium*. Se considera un reservorio de liberación lenta de diclorvos. El triclorfón se presenta en forma de solución concentrada emulsionable, polvos para disolución o aplicación en seco, gránulos, solución y soluciones concentradas de volumen muy reducido.

La concentración de triclorfón insecticida en el aire puede alcanzar 0,1 mg/m^3 al poco tiempo del rociamiento, pero a los pocos días los niveles se sitúan alrededor de 0,01 mg/m^3. En las aguas de escorrentía de zonas rociadas, la concentración de triclorfón puede alcanzar los 50 μg/litro; en cambio en las aguas de superficie suele ser mucho más baja y disminuye rápidamente.

El triclorfón se degrada rápidamente en el suelo; las concentraciones suelen disminuir hasta cantidades insignificantes durante el mes que sigue a la aplicación. Es relativamente estable en agua si el pH es inferior a 5,5; con un pH más elevado se transforma en diclorvos. Aunque los microorganismos y las plantas pueden metabolizar el triclorfón, la vía de eliminación más importante es la hidrólisis abiótica.

Salvo raras excepciones, las concentraciones de triclorfón en los cultivos son inferiores a 10 mg/kg al día siguiente de la aplicación, e inferiores a 0,1 mg/kg durante las dos semanas siguientes.

La leche de vacas tratadas con triclorfón para combatir plagas puede contener hasta 1,2 mg de residuos/litro a las dos horas de la aplicación, pero las cifras descienden hasta menos de 0,1 mg/litro a las 24 horas del tratamiento. No se han encontrado concentraciones importantes de este compuesto en la carne de animales tratados. En los huevos de gallinas tratadas se han comprobado valores de 0,05 mg de triclorfón/kg.

1.2 Ingestión, metabolismo y excreción

El triclorfón se absorbe fácilmente por todas las vías de exposición (oral, cutánea, respiratoria) y se distribuye rápidamente a los tejidos del cuerpo. Se detectaron concentraciones máximas en la sangre al cabo de 1-2 h, y la sustancia desapareció casi por completo del torrente sanguíneo en cuestión de 1,5-4 h. Se calculó que la semivida biológica del triclorfón en la sangre de mamíferos es de alrededor de 30 minutos.

Por deshidrocloración, el triclorfón se transforma en diclorvos (2,2-diclorovinil dimetil fosfato) en el agua y en los humores y tejidos de los seres vivos, si el pH es superior a 5,5. El diclorvos es la anticolinesterasa fisiológicamente activa. Las principales rutas de degradación son la desmetilación, la escisión del enlace P-C y la hidrólisis del éster con el diclorvos como producto intermediario. Los principales metabolitos del triclorfón que se encuentran *in vivo* son el demetil triclorfón, el demetil diclorvos, el dimetil hidrogenofosfato, el metil hidrogenofosfato, el ácido fosfórico y el tricloroetanol. El último metabolito se encuentra en la orina en forma de conjugado de glucurónido.

El triclorfón y sus productos metabólicos se eliminan principalmente con la orina. Los estudios realizados con triclorfón radiomarcado (^{14}C-metilo y ^{32}P-metilo) revelaron que la mayor parte de la sustancia se eliminaba en forma hidrosoluble, y una pequeña parte en forma soluble en cloroformo. Alrededor del 66%-70% de los productos hidrosolubles aparecían en la orina al cabo de 12 horas, mientras que el 24% del material marcado con ^{14}C-metilo se eliminaba en el aire espirado en forma de dióxido de carbono (CO_2). Se han detectado concentraciones bajas de triclorfón y sus metabolitos en la leche de bóvidos tras el tratamiento de éstos por vía oral y cutánea.

1.3 Efectos en organismos del medio ambiente

El triclorfón es moderadamente tóxico para los peces (los valores de la CL_{50} a las 96 h varían entre 0,45 mg/litro y 51 mg/litro) y de toxicidad moderada a elevada para los artrópodos acuáticos (la CL_{50} a las 48 h/96 h varía entre 0,75 μg/litro y 7800 μg/litro). En cambio, los valores observados en aguas de superficie tras aplicar el compuesto en bosques a razón de 6 kg/ha quedan por debajo de estos límites. Así pues, si es objeto de un uso normal, el triclorfón tendrá un efecto muy reducido o nulo en las poblaciones de organismos acuáticos, puesto que otros grupos como los moluscos y los microorganismos, son menos sensibles que los artrópodos. Los valores de la DL_{50} obtenidos en estudios de laboratorio (de 40 a 180 mg/kg) indican que este compuesto es moderadamente tóxico para las aves. En cambio, en estudios de campo no se observó efecto alguno en la población total, el número de parejas en época de cría, la viabilidad de los nidos ni la mortalidad de las aves canoras de los bosques tratados mediante aplicaciones aéreas del insecticida. Se observó cierta disminución de la actividad canora y mayor actividad de búsqueda de alimento, tal vez por haberse reducido las poblaciones de los organismos de que se nutren. Nada indica que el triclorfón perjudique a los organismos terrestres excepto los artrópodos. No se dispone de información sobre sus efectos en artrópodos beneficiosos.

1.4 Efectos en animales de laboratorio y en sistemas de ensayo in vitro

El triclorfón es un insecticida moderadamente tóxico para los animales de laboratorio. Los valores de la DL_{50} para el producto técnico administrado por vía oral a éstos varían entre 400 y 800 mg/kg de peso corporal; en la rata, los valores de la DL_{50} cuando se administra por vía cutánea superan los 2000 mg/kg de peso corporal.

La intoxicación por este compuesto origina los signos colinérgicos comúnmente relacionados con los organofosfatos y que se atribuyen a la acumulación de acetilcolina en las terminaciones nerviosas.

Se ha demostrado que el triclorfón técnico es moderadamente irritante para los ojos de la rata, aunque no para la piel del conejo. Se ha observado potencial de sensibilización cutánea en conejillos de Indias.

Se llevaron a cabo estudios de corto plazo sobre toxicidad por vía oral en ratas, perros, monos, conejos y conejillos de Indias. En uno de 16 semanas en ratas, en otro de 4 años en perros y en un tercero de 26 semanas en monos, se registraron respectivamente las siguientes concentraciones sin efectos observados (NOEL): 100 mg/kg de ración alimenticia, 50 mg/kg de ración alimenticia y 0,2 mg/kg de peso corporal (calculados respecto de la actividad de la colinesterasa en plasma, eritrocitos o encéfalo). La exposición de ratas por inhalación durante más de tres semanas indicó una NOEL de 12,7 mg/m^3, calculados respecto de la inhibición de la actividad de la colinesterasa en plasma, eritrocitos y encéfalo. Se llevaron a cabo estudios de toxicidad/carcinogenicidad a largo plazo en ratones, ratas, monos y hámsters tras la administración oral, intraperitoneal o cutánea. Se observaron efectos adversos en las gónadas de ratones y ratas expuestos por vía oral a 30 mg/kg de peso corporal y 400 mg/kg de ración alimenticia, respectivamente. En un estudio de 24 meses en ratas y otro de 10 años en monos, se determinaron valores de NOEL de 50 mg/kg de ración alimentaria y de 0,2 mg/kg de peso corporal, respectivamente. Los datos disponibles no aportan pruebas de carcinogenicidad tras la exposición prolongada de animales de laboratorio por diversas vías de administración.

Se ha comunicado que, en condiciones fisiológicas, el triclorfón tiene la propiedad de alquilizar al ADN. Los ensayos de mutagenicidad han dado resultados tanto positivos como negativos. Es posible que el diclorvos sea la causa, parcial o totalmente, de los efectos observados. La mayoría de los estudios de mutagenicidad *in vitro* en células tanto bacterianas como de mamíferos dieron resultado positivo; en cambio, pocos de los estudios *in vivo* dieron ese resultado.

Investigaciones realizadas en el ratón, la rata y el hámster indican que, en dosis lo bastante elevadas como para producir toxicidad materna, el triclorfón produce una respuesta teratógena en ratas. La exposición de ratas gestantes a dosis de 145 mg/kg de ración alimenticia provocó malformaciones fetales. La administración oral forzada de 400 mg/kg de peso corporal a hámsters produjo también toxicidad materna y respuesta teratógena. Por esta vía, la dosis más baja que produjo efectos teratógenos en la rata fue de 80 mg/kg de peso corporal. Los efectos son específicos según el momento del periodo de gestación en que se ingiere el producto. En este estudio de administración oral forzada se obtuvo una NOEL de 8 mg/kg.

En ratas y hámsters se han encontrado, respectivamente, NOEL de 8 mg/kg de peso corporal y 200 mg/kg de peso corporal. También se han comunicado respuestas teratógenas que afectaban al sistema nervioso central en el cerdo y el conejillo de Indias.

En cambio, no se observaron efectos teratógenos en un estudio de reproducción en tres generaciones de ratas, en el que con dosis elevadas se indujeron efectos reproductivos adversos. La NOEL en este estudio fue de 300 mg/kg de ración alimenticia.

Con dosis muy elevadas se han producido efectos neurotóxicos en animales.

En los mamíferos, el producto activo de la transformación es el diclorvos, cuya actividad como anticolinesterasa es como mínimo 100 veces mayor que la del triclorfón.

1.5 Efectos en el ser humano

Se han producido varios casos de envenenamiento agudo por exposición intencional (suicidio) o accidental. Los signos y síntomas de la intoxicación fueron los característicos de la inhibición de la acetilcolinesterasa: agotamiento, debilidad, confusión, sudación y salivación excesivas, dolores abdominales, vómitos, pupilas puntiformes y espasmos musculares. En casos graves se observaron pérdida de la consciencia y convulsiones, y la muerte se produjo en general por fallo respiratorio. En las víctimas que sobrevivieron gracias a la intervención médica, a veces se observó una polineuropatía diferida, acompañada de debilidad de los miembros inferiores, la cual apareció algunas semanas después de la exposición. En los casos mortales, la autopsia reveló alteraciones isquémicas en el encéfalo, la médula espinal y los ganglios vegetativos, lesiones de la vaina mielínica en la médula espinal y los pedúnculos cerebrales, y cambios estructurales en los axones de los nervios periféricos.

Se han producido algunos casos de envenenamiento ocupacional, principalmente por no observar las normas de seguridad. La exposición en un lugar de trabajo con concentraciones en el aire superiores a 0,5 mg/m^3 ocasionó la disminución de la colinesterasa plasmática y cambios del trazado electroencefalográfico. No obstante, estos signos desaparecieron por completo al cesar la exposición. No se ha comunicado ningún caso de sensibilización cutánea.

Este compuesto se ha usado extensamente para tratar la esquistosomiasis del ser humano. La administración de una dosis única (7-12 mg/kg) inhibió entre el 40 y el 60% de la colinesterasa del plasma y los eritrocitos, sin que aparecieran síntomas colinérgicos. En cambio, se observaron síntomas leves en personas tratadas con dosis repetidas. Las dosis elevadas (24 mg/kg) produjeron síntomas colinérgicos graves.

2. Conclusiones

- El insecticida triclorfón es un éster organofosforado moderadamente tóxico. La exposición excesiva que puede producirse al fabricarlo o utilizarlo y la ingestión accidental o intencional pueden provocar envenenamientos graves.

- La exposición de la población general al triclorfón se produce principalmente como resultado de las prácticas agrícolas y veterinarias y del tratamiento de la infestación por *Schistosoma haematobium.*

- Las ingestas de triclorfón comunicadas se encuentran muy por debajo de la ingesta diaria admisible establecida por la FAO/OMS y en principio no constituyen un riesgo para la salud de la población general.

- Si se siguen prácticas correctas de trabajo, medidas higiénicas y precauciones de seguridad, es poco probable que el triclorfón represente un riesgo para las personas expuestas por su trabajo.

- A pesar de su gran toxicidad para otros artrópodos que no se pretende destruir, el triclorfón se ha utilizado con escasos o nulos efectos adversos para las poblaciones de organismos del medio ambiente.

3. Recomendaciones

- Para proteger la salud de los trabajadores y de la población general, la manipulación y la aplicación del triclorfón deben encomendarse solamente a operarios bien supervisados y adiestrados, que observarán medidas adecuadas de seguridad y utilizarán el insecticida siguiendo prácticas correctas.

- La fabricación, la formulación, el uso agrícola y la evacuación del triclorfón deben sujetarse a una gestión cuidadosa para reducir al mínimo la contaminación del medio, en particular las aguas de superficie.

- Las poblaciones de trabajadores y de personas regularmente expuestos deben someterse a exámenes médicos periódicos.

- Las tasas de aplicación del triclorfón deben limitarse a fin de evitar efectos sobre artrópodos que no se pretende combatir. Este insecticida nunca debe rociarse sobre masas ni corrientes de agua.